Achieving Rural Health Equity and Well-Being

PROCEEDINGS OF A WORKSHOP

Steve Olson and Karen M. Anderson, *Rapporteurs*

Roundtable on Population Health Improvement

Roundtable on the Promotion of Health Equity

Board on Population Health and Public Health Practice

Health and Medicine Division

The National Academies of
SCIENCES · ENGINEERING · MEDICINE

THE NATIONAL ACADEMIES PRESS
Washington, DC
www.nap.edu

THE NATIONAL ACADEMIES PRESS 500 Fifth Street, NW Washington, DC 20001

This activity was supported by contracts between the National Academy of Sciences and Aetna Foundation (15-1381); The California Endowment (20171618); General Electric; Health Resources and Services Administration (HHSH25034007T); Kaiser Permanente; The Kresge Foundation (R-1512-255471); New York State Health Foundation (15-03733); Robert Wood Johnson Foundation (73263); and U.S. Department of Health and Human Services (HHSP23337054). Any opinions, findings, conclusions, or recommendations expressed in this publication do not necessarily reflect the views of any organization or agency that provided support for the project.

International Standard Book Number-13: 978-0-309-46905-0
International Standard Book Number-10: 0-309-46905-8
Digital Object Identifier: https://doi.org/10.17226/24967

Additional copies of this publication are available for sale from the National Academies Press, 500 Fifth Street, NW, Keck 360, Washington, DC 20001; (800) 624-6242 or (202) 334-3313; http://www.nap.edu.

Printed in the United States of America

Suggested citation: National Academies of Sciences, Engineering, and Medicine. 2018. *Achieving rural health equity and well-being: Proceedings of a workshop*. Washington, DC: The National Academies Press. doi: https://doi.org/10.17226/24967.

The National Academies of
SCIENCES • ENGINEERING • MEDICINE

The **National Academy of Sciences** was established in 1863 by an Act of Congress, signed by President Lincoln, as a private, nongovernmental institution to advise the nation on issues related to science and technology. Members are elected by their peers for outstanding contributions to research. Dr. Marcia McNutt is president.

The **National Academy of Engineering** was established in 1964 under the charter of the National Academy of Sciences to bring the practices of engineering to advising the nation. Members are elected by their peers for extraordinary contributions to engineering. Dr. C. D. Mote, Jr., is president.

The **National Academy of Medicine** (formerly the Institute of Medicine) was established in 1970 under the charter of the National Academy of Sciences to advise the nation on medical and health issues. Members are elected by their peers for distinguished contributions to medicine and health. Dr. Victor J. Dzau is president.

The three Academies work together as the **National Academies of Sciences, Engineering, and Medicine** to provide independent, objective analysis and advice to the nation and conduct other activities to solve complex problems and inform public policy decisions. The National Academies also encourage education and research, recognize outstanding contributions to knowledge, and increase public understanding in matters of science, engineering, and medicine.

Learn more about the National Academies of Sciences, Engineering, and Medicine at **www.nationalacademies.org**.

PLANNING COMMITTEE ON ACHIEVING RURAL HEALTH EQUITY AND WELL-BEING[1]

JULIE A. BALDWIN, Center for Health Equity Research, Northern Arizona University
MARTHE GOLD, The New York Academy of Medicine
JEFFREY A. HENDERSON, Black Hills Center for American Indian Health
DENNIS JOHNSON, Children's Health Fund
OCTAVIO N. MARTINEZ, Hogg Foundation for Mental Health, The University of Texas at Austin
PHYLLIS D. MEADOWS, The Kresge Foundation
ALAN MORGAN, National Rural Health Association
TIM SIZE, Rural Wisconsin Health Cooperative

[1] The National Academies of Sciences, Engineering, and Medicine's planning committees are solely responsible for organizing the workshop, identifying topics, and choosing speakers. The responsibility for the published Proceedings of a Workshop rests with the workshop rapporteurs and the institution.

ROUNDTABLE ON POPULATION HEALTH IMPROVEMENT[1]

GEORGE J. ISHAM (*Co-Chair*), HealthPartners
SANNE MAGNAN (*Co-Chair*), University of Minnesota
PHILIP M. ALBERTI, Association of American Medical Colleges
TERRY ALLAN, Cuyahoga County Board of Health
JOHN AUERBACH, Trust for America's Health
CATHY BAASE, The Dow Chemical Company, Michigan Health Improvement Alliance
DEBBIE I. CHANG, Nemours
CHARLES J. FAZIO, HealthPartners
GEORGE R. FLORES, The California Endowment
KATHY GERWIG, Health and Wellness and Environmental Stewardship Officer, Kaiser Permanente
ALAN GILBERT, GE Healthymagination
MARY LOU GOEKE, United Way of Santa Cruz County
MARTHE GOLD, The New York Academy of Medicine
MARC N. GOUREVITCH, New York University Langone School of Medicine
GARTH GRAHAM, Aetna Foundation
GARY R. GUNDERSON, Wake Forest University
WAYNE JONAS, H&S Ventures
ROBERT M. KAPLAN, Stanford University
DAVID A. KINDIG, University of Wisconsin–Madison
PAULA M. LANTZ, University of Michigan
MICHELLE LARKIN, Robert Wood Johnson Foundation
THOMAS A. LAVEIST, The George Washington University
JEFFREY LEVI, The George Washington University
SARAH R. LINDE, Health Resources and Services Administration
SHARRIE McINTOSH, New York State Health Foundation
PHYLLIS D. MEADOWS, The Kresge Foundation
BOBBY MILSTEIN, Rethink Health
JOSÉ T. MONTERO, Office for State, Tribal, Local and Territorial Support, Centers for Disease Control and Prevention
MARY PITTMAN, Public Health Institute
PAMELA RUSSO, Robert Wood Johnson Foundation
JAMES N. WEINSTEIN, Dartmouth-Hitchcock

[1] The National Academies of Sciences, Engineering, and Medicine's forums and roundtables do not issue, review, or approve individual documents. The responsibility for the published Proceedings of a Workshop rests with the workshop rapporteurs and the institution.

Roundtable on Population Health Improvement Staff

ALINA BACIU, Director, Roundtable on Population Health Improvement
DARLA THOMPSON, Program Officer (through August 2017)
KIMANI HAMILTON-WRAY, Senior Program Assistant (from April 2017)
HOPE HARE, Administrative Assistant
ROSE MARIE MARTINEZ, Senior Director, Board on Population Health and Public Health Practice

ROUNDTABLE ON THE PROMOTION OF HEALTH EQUITY[1]

ANTONIA VILLARRUEL (*Chair*), University of Pennsylvania
PATRICIA BAKER, Connecticut Health Foundation
JULIE A. BALDWIN, Center for Health Equity Research, Northern Arizona University
GILLIAN BARCLAY, Nevada Governor's Office of Economic Development
NED CALONGE, The Colorado Trust
KENDALL M. CAMPBELL, Brody School of Medicine, East Carolina University
LUTHER T. CLARK, Merck & Co., Inc.
FRANCISCO GARCÍA, Pima County Department of Health
JEFFREY A. HENDERSON, Black Hills Center for American Indian Health
EVE J. HIGGINBOTHAM, University of Pennsylvania
CARA V. JAMES, Centers for Medicare & Medicaid Services
CHRIS KABEL, The Kresge Foundation
MELENIE MAGNOTTA, Aetna Foundation
OCTAVIO N. MARTINEZ, Hogg Foundation for Mental Health, The University of Texas at Austin
CHRISTINE RAMEY, Health Resources and Services Administration
MELISSA A. SIMON, Northwestern University Feinberg School of Medicine
PATTIE TUCKER, Centers for Disease Control and Prevention
UCHENNA S. UCHENDU, Office of Health Equity, U.S. Department of Veterans Affairs
ROHIT VARMA, University of Southern California
WINSTON WONG, Kaiser Permanente

Roundtable on the Promotion of Health Equity Staff

KAREN ANDERSON, Director, Roundtable on the Promotion of Health Equity
ANNA MARTIN, Senior Program Assistant
HOPE HARE, Administrative Assistant
ROSE MARIE MARTINEZ, Senior Director, Board on Population Health and Public Health Practice

---

[1] The National Academies of Sciences, Engineering, and Medicine's forums and roundtables do not issue, review, or approve individual documents. The responsibility for the published Proceedings of a Workshop rests with the workshop rapporteurs and the institution.

Reviewers

This Proceedings of a Workshop was reviewed in draft form by individuals chosen for their diverse perspectives and technical expertise. The purpose of this independent review is to provide candid and critical comments that will assist the National Academies of Sciences, Engineering, and Medicine in making each published proceedings as sound as possible and to ensure that it meets the institutional standards for quality, objectivity, evidence, and responsiveness to the charge. The review comments and draft manuscript remain confidential to protect the integrity of the process.

We thank the following individuals for their review of this proceedings:

CATHERINE BRYAN, First Nations Development Institute
ALAN MORGAN, National Rural Health Association
WALTER NILES, Office of Minority Health and Health Equity
GLENDA SMITH, University of Alabama

Although the reviewers listed above provided many constructive comments and suggestions, they were not asked to endorse the content of the proceedings nor did they see the final draft before its release. The review of this proceedings was overseen by **DEBORAH POWELL,** University of Minnesota. She was responsible for making certain that an independent examination of this proceedings was carried out in accordance with standards of the National Academies and that all review comments were carefully considered. Responsibility for the final content rests entirely with the rapporteurs and the National Academies.

Contents

1

Introduction[1]

Rural counties make up about 80 percent of the land area of the United States, but they contain less than 20 percent of the U.S. population (Ingram and Franco, 2012). The relative sparseness of the population in rural areas is one of many factors that influence the health and well-being of rural Americans. Rural areas have histories, economies, and cultures that differ from those of cities and from one rural area to another. Understanding these differences is critical to taking steps to improve health and well-being in rural areas and to reduce health disparities among rural populations.

To explore the impacts of economic, demographic, and social issues in rural communities and to learn about asset-based approaches to addressing the associated challenges, the Roundtable on Population Health Improvement and the Roundtable on the Promotion of Health Equity of the National Academies of Sciences, Engineering, and Medicine held a workshop titled "Achieving Rural Health Equity and Well-Being: Challenges and Opportunities" on June 13, 2017, in Prattville, Alabama, outside the city of Montgomery. The two roundtables brought complementary but distinct perspectives and expertise on the topic.

[1] The planning committee's role was limited to planning the workshop, and the Proceedings of a Workshop was prepared by the rapporteurs as a factual account of what occurred at the workshop. Statements, recommendations, and opinions expressed are those of individual presenters and participants and are not necessarily endorsed or verified by the National Academies of Sciences, Engineering, and Medicine. They should not be construed as reflecting any group consensus.

Since February 2013, the Roundtable on Population Health Improvement has been providing a trusted venue for leaders from the public and private sectors to meet and discuss the leverage points and opportunities arising from challenges and changes in the social and political environment for achieving better population health. The roundtable's vision is of a strong, healthful, and productive society that cultivates human capital and equal opportunity. This vision rests on the recognition that outcomes such as improved life expectancy, quality of life, and health for all are shaped by interdependent social, economic, environmental, genetic, behavioral, and health care factors, and that robust national and community-based policies and dependable resources are needed to achieve that vision.

The Roundtable on the Promotion of Health Equity serves as the conveners of the nation's experts in health disparities and health equity, with the goal of raising awareness and driving change. The roundtable was created in 2007 to promote health equity and reduce health disparities by advancing the visibility of and understanding about the inequities in health and health care among racial and ethnic populations, amplifying research, policy, and community-centered programs, and catalyzing the emergence of new leaders, partners, and stakeholders.

WORKSHOP OBJECTIVES

An important activity of the roundtables is to hold workshops for their members, stakeholders, and the public to discuss issues that contribute to eliminating disparities and improving the nation's health. An independent planning committee, comprising Julie Baldwin, Marthe Gold, Jeffrey Henderson, Dennis Johnson, Octavio Martinez, Phyllis Meadows, Alan Morgan, and Tim Size, was charged with developing a workshop to explore how rural communities in different parts of the United States handle the challenges and opportunities of advancing health equity and well-being (see Box 1-1). The workshop was designed to do the following:

- Explore impacts of economic issues, immigration, and racial inequities in U.S. rural communities
- Learn about asset-based approaches to addressing these challenges

To achieve these objectives, the planning committee organized panels that revolved around how regional philanthropic organizations leverage resources to help address unique local and regional needs, how local finance and community advocacy organizations work to create the conditions for economic prosperity, and how health sector institutions work to ensure access to quality health care services for rural communities.

BOX 1-1
Statement of Task

An ad hoc committee will plan and implement a 1-day public workshop that will explore initiatives focused on improving community well-being. Particular attention will be paid to the intersecting challenges of racism, structural inequities, and poverty in the context of rural geographic regions. The workshop may include invited presentations on, and discussion of, initiatives created to tackle systematic disinvestment in rural communities, implications for improving the social determinants of health (e.g., jobs, economy, education, transportation, affordable housing), and access to and quality of health care services. The workshop is intended to illustrate some promising and constructive actions that rural communities facing these enormous challenges are taking to equitably improve residents' health and well-being. The committee will plan and organize the workshop. A proceedings of the presentations and discussion at the workshop will be prepared by a designated rapporteur in accordance with institutional guidelines.

ORGANIZATION AND THEMES OF THE WORKSHOP

This Proceedings of a Workshop synthesizes the discussions held at the workshop, highlights the speakers' perspectives on rural health equity and well-being, and provides an overview of showcased initiatives and approaches to meeting the particular challenges and opportunities in improving health in rural communities. Chapter 2 summarizes two keynote presentations that provided an overview of differences between rural and urban communities and the challenges and opportunities rural communities face. Chapter 3 summarizes presentations on the strengths and resources that rural communities have and the ways in which local and regional foundations can build on those strengths. Chapter 4 examines in greater detail some of the factors that contribute to health disparities in rural areas, including economic, historical, and cultural forces. The presentations outlined in Chapter 5 focus on a range of communities, including rural Alabamians, people living along the U.S.–Mexico border, and people living near rural hospitals that close, and consider different ways to overcome the unique challenges in rural communities. Chapter 6 provides the final comments and reflections on the day's presentations (see Box 1-2 for highlights).

In accordance with the policies of the National Academies, workshop participants did not attempt to establish any conclusions or recommendations about needs and future directions, focusing instead on issues discussed by the speakers and workshop participants. In addition, the

BOX 1-2
Highlights and Main Points of Final Reflections Made by Individual Speakers

- The history of rural America is an integral part of the history of the United States. Both have been shaped by how the nation was formed, the influence of slavery and the confiscation of land, and the struggle against oppression. It is a living history, and America is a changing land. (Wong)
- Rural inequities are a superb example of the intersectionality of the factors that contribute to disparities. It is bad to be poor, even worse to be poor and a person of color, and even worse to be poor and a person of color, undocumented, living in a rural area with limited educational opportunities, and no access to transportation. We need to consider the whole person and the intersectionality of inequities when we think about how to address inequity. (Calonge)
- The social determinants of health and [available] assets and resources can differ between urban and rural areas. Understanding and changing these root causes of disparities can help reduce those disparities. (Isham)
- Poverty plays an overwhelming role in generating challenges in rural communities. (Baase)
- The sparseness of the population in rural communities can make it more difficult than in urban areas to gather data and expand programs that address health disparities. (Gourevitch)
- Despite their differences, many of the problems rural and urban areas face are similar, including problems of access, transportation, and education. The commonality of problems creates an opportunity for shared approaches to solutions. (Villarruel)
- Rural clinics, federally qualified health centers, community health workers, and telehealth are especially suited for rural areas. Because of the role of poverty, linkages with people working on economic and community development can be particularly important. (Pittman)

planning committee's role was limited to planning the workshop. The Proceedings of a Workshop was prepared by the workshop rapporteurs Steve Olson and Karen Anderson as a factual summary of what occurred at the workshop.

2

Potential Challenges and Opportunities in Rural Communities

Points Made by the Speakers

- Inequities based on race and ethnicity overlap with and intensify inequities based on geography. (Meit)
- Across most of the social determinants of health, rural populations do not fare as well as urban populations. (Meit)
- Solutions to problems that work in urban areas may not work in rural areas. (Morris)
- History and culture are assets for rural communities and can be leveraged to improve health outcomes. (Meit)
- Rural health and inequities between rural and urban areas have traditionally been bipartisan issues. (Morris)

Rural America is not a smaller version of urban America, observed Tom Morris, associate administrator in the Federal Office of Rural Health Policy in the Health Resources and Services Administration (HRSA) of the U.S. Department of Health and Human Services (HHS), in the first of two keynote presentations at the workshop (see Figure 2-1). On average, rural areas have higher levels of poverty, higher percentages of older adults, and slower growing or declining populations. Morris explained that the payer mix for health care tends to be different than what is found in urban areas. In rural communities, Medicare, Medicaid, and the Children's Health Insurance Program are the dominant payers. In

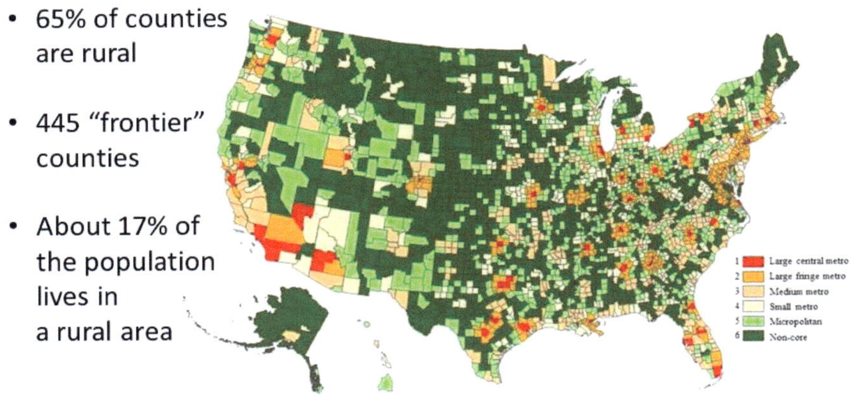

FIGURE 2-1 Land area in the United States classified as rural.
SOURCES: As presented by Tom Morris, June 13, 2017; Ingram and Franco, 2012.

urban areas, third-party insurance tends to be the dominant payer. As a result, changes to Medicare and Medicaid have a disproportionate effect on rural providers and their ability to provide care to the citizens in their communities.

Although there are commonalities among rural areas, they can also differ greatly from each other. Rural areas in the deep South face different issues than rural areas in Maine, Morris pointed out. In the western United States, weather can be a limiting factor in a way that it is not in other parts of the country. The mix of health care providers varies, although many areas suffer from provider shortages.

Multiple definitions of the term *rural* exist. The Office of Management and Budget (OMB) uses a system based on counties. The Census Bureau uses a system based on census tracts. In his presentation, Morris used OMB's definition, which identifies about 17 percent of the population as living in rural areas spread across about 80 percent of the country's land mass (see Figure 2-1). About two-thirds of the nation's approximately 3,100 counties and county equivalents are rural, including about 450 geographically remote and isolated "frontier" counties.

Nonmetropolitan areas have fewer physicians than metropolitan areas—5.5 versus 7.9 per 10,000 people (Larson et al., 2016). When nurse practitioners and physician assistants are included, the disparities remain—11.6 versus 16.2 per 10,000 people. The same applies to dentists—3.6 versus 5.9 per 10,000 people—and to dental hygienists—4.5 versus 5.0 per 10,000 people.

Even more striking, said Morris, is the relative lack of mental health providers in rural communities. About 200 counties—17 percent of the nonmetropolitan counties—have no mental health practitioner at all: "No psychologists, no psychiatrists, no licensed clinical social workers, no psychiatric nurse practitioners," he explained. This is a "real challenge," said Morris, for addressing behavioral health.

Given the economic challenge of providing care in rural communities, federal legislation provides special protections to the hospital and clinical infrastructure in these areas. Of the approximately 2,000 rural hospitals in the United States (out of a total of 5,000 to 6,000 hospitals, depending on definitions), approximately 1,300 are "critical access hospitals," meaning that they have 25 beds or fewer and, in most cases, are more than 35 miles from another hospital. These hospitals get special protection from Medicare and an eased regulatory burden. Without these protections, said Morris, the United States would potentially have "a real problem in terms of ensuring access to inpatient and emergency care in rural communities."

Over the past 15 years, the system of federally qualified health centers (FQHCs) in the United States has grown substantially, with a particular emphasis on oral health and mental health. About 10,000 FQHC service sites are scattered across the United States, with about 40 percent of these either located in or serving rural communities. In addition, about 4,000 Medicare-certified rural health clinics exist in the United States. About half of these are provider based, meaning that they are owned by small, rural hospitals.

From 1999 to about 2010, the critical access hospital designation had stabilized rural hospitals' economic challenges, according to Morris. However, since 2010, about 79 rural hospitals have closed their doors or suspended operations (although, as of the middle of 2017, only two had closed in that year).[1] Several factors account for these closures, including declining populations, declining in-patient use, and changes in the payer mix, said Morris. "It is tough to keep a full-service hospital open in some communities where you just don't have enough population base," said Morris. In other cases, "market factors [are] at work that made it impossible for those facilities to continue." (The section titled "The Closure of Rural Hospitals" in Chapter 5 discusses this issue in more detail.)

In rural areas, emergency medical services (EMS) are largely volunteer driven and have to cover vast geographic areas with a low patient volume. "Providing EMS can be a real challenge," said Morris. In addition, rural public health departments derive less of their revenue from local communities and are more reliant on billing for services than their urban counterparts.

[1] As of the workshop date, there were 70; this is a continuously fluctuating number.

The differences between rural and urban areas create several pitfalls for federal health care policy, Morris observed. Payment systems are based on the average cost of cases, but in rural areas a high-cost case paired with a fixed-cost payment can create economic difficulties. Solutions to problems that work in urban areas may not work in rural areas. For example, when Medicare started paying for diabetes self-education management, many rural communities could not meet the requirements for trained personnel needed for reimbursement. While this situation "has gotten better over the years," said Morris, "I offer it more as a metaphor for some of the challenges when we think about this." Even the very successful Nurse–Family Partnership program has requirements that are not necessarily attainable for smaller communities in terms of the credentials of the care team required to implement the model, he commented.

As discussions about the prospect of federal funding move toward block grants, states may focus on the areas with highest needs, in part to meet performance metrics, while overlooking low-population areas, Morris continued. Other kinds of grants also may focus on areas that contain larger numbers of people, and evaluations may pass over rural areas because the population base is not large enough for statistically significant results. "I am all for academic rigor, but there are ways to think differently about evaluation so as not to let it be at the detriment of a high-need population," he said.

Technological approaches, such as telehealth, are often held out as solutions for rural health care. But technology is a tool, not a solution, said Morris. There are still challenges in fully integrating telehealth into the day-to-day delivery of care. Similarly, electronic health records (EHRs) provide the potential for clinical information to follow the rural patients who get care in urban settings, but these systems continue to have gaps owing to challenges with interoperability and health information exchange. In addition, some parts of the country still do not have access to robust or affordable broadband service, which limits the flow of information.

FEDERAL ACTIONS

The federal government invests in rural health through a number of mechanisms, Morris observed, including the following:

- Workforce training
- Clinician placement, including through the National Health Service Corps
- Infrastructure support
- Targeting resources by designating shortage areas
- Enhanced payments through Medicare and Medicaid

- Pilots and demonstrations
- Provision and support of public coverage
- Investments in technology, including telehealth, broadband, and EHRs

A range of federal agencies support these efforts, such as when the U.S. Department of Agriculture helps rebuild or renovate a hospital or a community health center, or the Federal Communications Commission supports broad communications infrastructure [that also meets health sector needs]. The federal government also significantly improves health care delivery in rural areas through Medicare, Medicaid, and other forms of allocation and direct funding.

The Office of Rural Health Policy under HRSA was created about 30 years ago to be the voice of rural health in HHS. It reviews how federal policies and programs affect rural communities and seeks to put research findings into the hands of leaders in both rural and urban areas at the state and federal levels. It funds seven rural health research centers around the country and a national clearinghouse for rural health information at the University of North Dakota. It is "trying to develop a rural evidence base so that people can replicate what we know works in rural communities," said Morris.

The office invests about $60 million per year in community-based funding that is limited to rural communities so they do not have to compete with metropolitan areas. Its programs include public health screening, care coordination, defibrillator and opioid-reversal programs, grants focused on performance and quality improvement for small rural hospitals, state offices of rural health, telehealth network grants and resource centers, and licensure and portability efforts. As an example, Morris cited a brief prepared by the National Advisory Committee on Rural Health and Human Services (2017) on the social determinants of health in a rural context. One of the committee's key findings was that funding mechanisms can make it difficult for rural communities to bring resources to bear on health disparities, and the committee offered several recommendations to overcome these difficulties.

Morris explained that in fiscal year 2016, 160,000 parents and children nationwide received HRSA-supported home visiting services. These services took place in 35 percent of all urban counties and 23 percent of all rural counties. Training grants support more than 187,000 students from rural areas, and HRSA-supported training spots include about 8,400 rural locations.

Other parts of HHS are relevant to rural health, including the Agency for Healthcare Research and Quality, the Administration for Children and Families, the Centers for Medicare & Medicaid Services (CMS), the

National Institutes of Health, the Substance Abuse and Mental Health Services Administration, the Centers for Disease Control and Prevention (CDC), the Indian Health Service, and the Administration for Community Living. For example, the Health Rural Council within CMS has helped that part of HHS understand the challenges of rural communities. CMS has also supported Innovation Center awards, technical assistance targeted to rural and underserved areas, and the Connected Care Management Campaign, which is focused on patients with one or more chronic health conditions, including patients in rural and underserved areas. CDC has run a series of articles on rural health in its *Morbidity and Mortality Weekly Report*. "It is great that CDC is now looking at rural health. That is the kind of thing that needs to happen," said Morris. "They are, in my mind, the key public health agency in HHS, and when they focus on rural health issues, it garners national attention," he said.

At an interagency level, the Federal Interagency Health Equity Team has considered rural issues. The National Advisory Committee on Rural Health and Human Services focuses on both rural health and rural human service issues, issues policy briefs, and makes recommendations to the HHS secretary. In addition, federal agencies invest in non–health care services that have an effect on health, Morris pointed out in response to a question. For example, the Center for Innovation at CMS has supported the Accountable Health Communities Model, which focuses on services such as housing that affect health outcomes.

OVERLAPPING INEQUITIES

Inequities based on race and ethnicity overlap with and intensify inequities based on geography, observed Michael Meit, co-director of the NORC Walsh Center for Rural Health Analysis and senior fellow in NORC at The University of Chicago Public Health Research Department, in the second keynote address of the workshop. "When you overlay those two, you have a dual disparity. That is where you will find many of the greatest disparities we have in our country," he said.

Meit explained that on average, life expectancies in rural areas are lower than those in urban areas, and the gap has been widening since the two rates were equal in the early 1980s (see Figure 2-2). Other recent data (not shown in Figure 2-2) reveal that for the U.S. population as a whole, life expectancy has recently declined for the first time since the AIDS epidemic of the early 1990s. The current decline in life expectancy is tied to three "diseases of despair," said Meit: overdose (including opioids), alcoholic liver disease, and suicide. These conditions are disproportionately affecting rural populations, Meit added, further widening the gap between urban and rural.

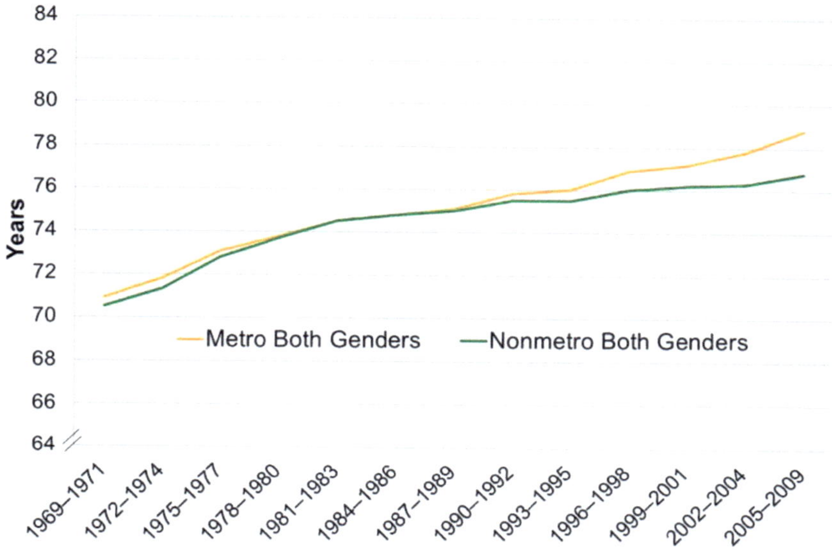

FIGURE 2-2 Average life expectancy at birth.
SOURCES: As presented by Michael Meit, June 13, 2017; adapted from Singh and Siahpush, 2014.

More broadly, social factors have a major effect on health, Meit observed. The Healthy People 2020 Framework divided the social determinants of health into five categories:

1. Economic stability—poverty, employment, food security, housing stability
2. Education—high school graduation, enrollment in higher education, language and literacy, early childhood education and development
3. Social and community context—social cohesion, civic participation, perceptions of discrimination and equity, incarceration/institutionalization
4. Health and health care—access to health care, access to primary care, health literacy
5. Neighborhood and built environment—access to healthy foods, quality of housing, crime and violence, environmental conditions

Across most of these social determinants of health, rural populations do not fare as well as urban populations. The median household income in rural areas is $10,000 less per year on average than in urban areas, said Meit. About 5 percent more children live in poverty in rural counties (26 percent) than in urban counties (21 percent). In rural counties, 16.5 percent of adults have less than a high school education (compared with 14.7 percent in urban counties), 36.3 percent have only a high school diploma (compared with 31.9 percent in urban counties), and 17.4 percent have a bachelor's degree or higher (compared with 24 percent in urban counties), Meit explained.

In his presentation, Meit focused on the approximately 350 counties in the United States designated as "persistent poverty counties," where the county has had a greater than 20 percent rate of poverty since the 1980 census (see Figure 2-3). "Don't think that this is the only place where poverty lives, but this is where poverty is persistent," noted Meit. The counties are largely rural, including counties in Appalachia, the Mississippi Delta, the "Stroke Belt" in the southeastern United States, and along the U.S.–Mexico border.

These regions are also the areas with the highest rural minority populations, with African Americans in the South and Southeast, Hispanics

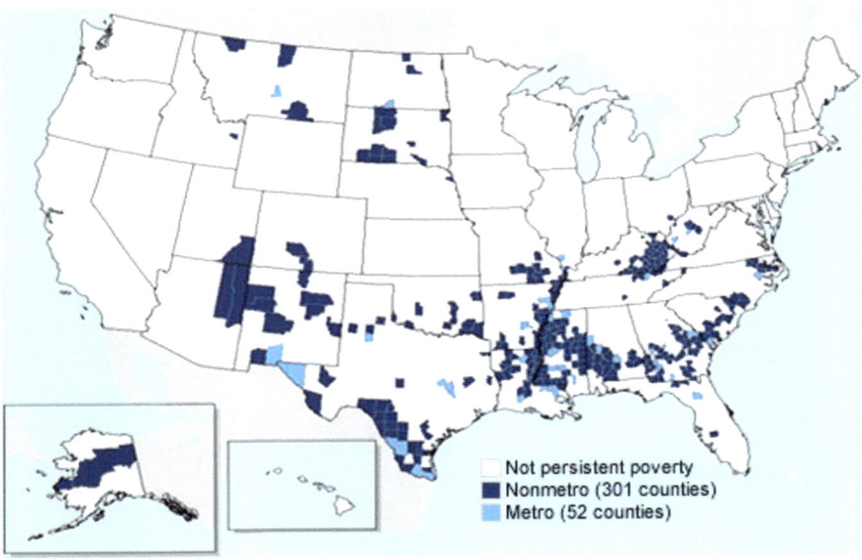

FIGURE 2-3 Persistent poverty counties have had poverty rates of at least 20 percent in the U.S. censuses of 1980, 1990, and 2000 and in the American Community Survey 5-year estimates of 2007–2011.
SOURCES: As presented by Michael Meit, June 13, 2017; USDA, 2017.

along the border, and Native Americans in New Mexico, Arizona, and the Plains states. In addition, these counties are often designated as Health Professional Shortage Areas (HPSAs). The connecting link, said Meit, is poverty, which "is probably the greatest predictor of health status that we have."

A study done through the Rural Health Reform Policy Research Center, a collaborative effort of the NORC Walsh Center for Rural Health and the University of North Dakota Center for Rural Health, examined the effect of rurality on mortality and regional differences in the primary and underlying causes of death. The study examined mortality data for the 10 leading causes of death by age bracket (for the 25 to 64 years age range, this included cerebrovascular diseases, diabetes, heart disease, homicide, liver diseases, lower respiratory diseases, malignant neoplasms, septicemia, suicide, and unintentional injuries). Data were analyzed for each of the 10 regions into which HHS divides the country (with the addition of the Appalachian and Delta regions separately), and the National Center for Health Statistics' urban–rural classification scheme for counties (which distinguishes large central, large fringe, small/medium metropolitan, micropolitan, and noncore) was applied to the analyses along with age and gender (although not race or ethnicity).

In region 4, which covers the southeastern United States and includes a high percentage of African Americans, men ages 25 to 64 living in rural counties generally fare far worse on measures of the 10 leading causes of death than those living in urban counties, with the exception of homicides, said Meit. Rural women living in rural counties fare worse on all 10 leading causes of death. Rural men in this region are more than twice as likely to die from lower respiratory disease as other men in the United States, and 60 percent more likely to die from unintentional injury. Rural women in this region are more than 2.2 times as likely to die from lower respiratory disease, twice as likely to die from unintentional injury, and 60 percent more likely to die from diabetes.

In region 6, which covers Arkansas, Louisiana, New Mexico, Oklahoma, and Texas, and has a high percentage of Hispanics, a similar pattern appears, with lower respiratory diseases and unintentional injuries especially prominent among rural men and women. Similar conclusions can be drawn about regions that have large numbers of Native Americans. Rural health indicators are especially poor where rural areas intersect with large minority populations, Meit said.

Every part of the country "has a story to tell," said Meit. It may be a story about slavery, about the creation of Indian reservations, or about cross-border relations, but these stories reflect both historical processes and current health status. "You cannot separate [disparities] from culture and history. That is something we need to delve into much more deeply," he explained.

Meit also focused on the Appalachian region, a region that faces considerable health disparities despite not having large minority populations. Meit discussed what have been referred to as the "diseases of despair," which include deaths resulting from overdose, suicide, and alcoholic liver disease. In the Appalachian region, mortality rates for liver disease, suicide, and unintentional injuries (which include overdose deaths) are all above the national average for men ages 25 to 64. Rates for rural women are also above the national average for suicide and unintentional injuries.

Recent work conducted by the NORC Walsh Center for Rural Health Analysis, on behalf of the Appalachian Regional Commission, has shown that the combined age-adjusted mortality rate for diseases of despair in Appalachia is 66.6 per 100,000 people, compared with 48.6 per 100,000 people in the United States as a whole—including a 7 percent higher rate of mortality resulting from alcoholic liver disease, a 17 percent higher rate of mortality resulting from suicide, and a 40 percent higher rate of mortality resulting from overdose deaths (69 percent of which is attributable to opioid overdose). Future analyses will explore patterns within Appalachia by age, subregion, and county economic indicators, said Meit.

Meit ended by talking about some of the resources available to strengthen rural health programs. The NORC Walsh Center is developing a series of evidence-based toolkits based on what works in rural communities. Most programs are not tested in rural communities, and these communities may need unique models, said Meit. The toolkits capture programs that work in rural areas and help communities replicate those models, with new toolkits being created on a continuing basis. Toolkits are housed in the Community Health Gateway, part of the Rural Health Information Hub, which Meit referred to as "a one-stop shop for everything rural."

Meit also highlighted new work being conducted by the NORC Walsh Center that is funded by the Robert Wood Johnson Foundation. This body of work seeks to identify strengths and opportunities that can accelerate and improve health and well-being in rural communities; identify factors (and partners) that can influence health and well-being within rural communities, such as transportation, faith, education, and business; and identify opportunities for action and a set of recommendations for diverse rural stakeholders and funders. Through this project, the NORC Walsh Center has worked to identify assets that can be leveraged in rural communities, including individual, organizational, community, and cultural assets (Kretzmann and McKnight, 1993). Meit noted that the cultural assets are an important component of this framework in rural communities, describing them as "the greatest assets that we have." He concluded:

> People are proud of their heritage. They are proud of their communities. . . . Rural communities are close-knit. People know each other. They come to each other's aid. They are resilient. There are a lot of really positive factors about being in a rural community that can be leveraged.

DISCUSSION

In a wide-ranging discussion session, Morris and Meit touched on a number of issues, including scope of practice, the Patient Protection and Affordable Care Act (ACA), public health programs in rural areas, and the politics of health care.

In response to a question about state policies on scope of practice for advanced practice nurses, Morris pointed out that primary care providers "should be able to practice to the extent of their training." But these issues are inevitably political, he said, adding that "the best thing we can do is bring attention to it." For example, the National Conference of State Legislatures published on its website a state-by-state comparison of scope of practice for various health care professionals.

Both speakers also commented on the ACA, for which Congress was considering a replacement at the time of the workshop. Meit pointed out that many people gained insurance under the act, but they did not necessarily gain access. Demand for health care increased, but the demand was often directed toward health departments that already had provider shortages.

Morris took a longer-term view by citing the history of Medicare Part D, which increased access to medicines. As the program evolved, it garnered broad bipartisan support. He also pointed out, however, that insurance regulation tends to work against rural communities. Risk needs to be pooled among larger populations, he said, to attract insurers, "and not just for the Affordable Care marketplaces but for every form of insurance."

In response to a question about the training of EMS personnel, Morris observed that they are volunteers, which raises questions about the requirements they can be asked to meet. Yet, even a little training in behavioral health care "would go a long way," he said. One positive model is the concept of community paramedicine (i.e., paramedics and emergency medical technicians operate in expanded roles),[2] in which rural communities ask how they can deploy the resources they have in a more efficient and effective manner. If a reimbursement system can be

---

[2] From Rural Health Information Hub: https://www.ruralhealthinfo.org/topics/community-paramedicine (accessed November 20, 2017).

worked out, such a model could accommodate wellness checks, home visits, and other services.

Meit reemphasized the need for federal dollars to make it to rural areas in an equitable way. States tend to focus on larger population centers to produce results that justify the expenses. "That also means, as a byproduct, that dollars aren't making it to rural communities, which are facing very significant disparities," he said, adding that a possible policy proposal would be to call for ensuring that the same percentage of federal funding for such purposes be allocated to rural communities as the percentage of a state's population in rural areas.

Workshop participant Dale Quinney, executive director of the Alabama Rural Health Association, pointed to several problems with definitions of "rural" areas. The diagram of chronic poverty counties in Alabama included Pickens, Hale, and Lowndes counties as urban, but "there ain't no way that those are urban," he said. The Census Bureau asks states for input on the categorization of census tracts, but that does not happen with counties. Similarly, the methodology for specifying HPSAs is flawed, he said. Yet, HPSAs are associated with physician incentives that can skew decisions about whether or not to provide care in a particular place. "We had a county not long ago that was about to lose its HPSA status because it employed one physician too many," said Quinney. "Physicians threatened to leave and go elsewhere because they were going to lose that bonus payment each year." Incentives should work to reward rather than punish the provision of more care, he argued.

In response to a question about the role of public health in rural areas, Meit observed that every state has a unique public health infrastructure. Some state health departments include their Medicaid agencies. Others include environmental programs. Some state health departments are centralized while others are decentralized. This makes it difficult to quantify the public health infrastructure in states and even harder to compare funding among states, he said.

Overall, however, the public health infrastructure "struggles more in our rural communities," Meit continued, adding "We have good data to demonstrate that." Furthermore, funding seems to be getting even tighter for small rural health departments. Meit asked:

> What is the implication of not having boots on the ground in our communities to do disease surveillance, to track infectious disease, to do epidemiological investigations to control outbreaks, to do health education, all of the core work of public health?

Public health organizations and associations have tended to overlook rural issues, and the National Rural Health Association has not done a great job of talking about public health, said Meit, adding:

> They have tried over the years, but their membership is largely hospitals and clinics, so they talk about access. The public health organizations tend to have more urban membership, so they don't talk about rural. We need to bring this all together and talk about rural population health. That is the path forward.

Morris added that the federal agencies working on human service rural infrastructure, such as the Administration for Children and Families and the Administration for Community Living, are even more stretched than the health agencies. Yet jobs, economic sustainability, and families are critical factors in health issues.

In a discussion about the dissemination and scaling up of successful models, Morris pointed out that it is often easier to ramp up a model that has proven successful in a rural area than to translate an evidence-based model from an urban area to a rural one, given the frequent need to discard parts of the model for use in a rural area. Rural communities can be better places to test models than urban communities because fewer things are going on that can potentially influence outcomes.

Rural communities also have more room for improvement, said Morris, and a lack of resources can lead to more innovation in rural communities than urban ones. He explained:

> When you don't have a lot of dollars coming in, you have to be creative in thinking about how you get things done. If we can capture that and figure out what is it that can be distilled and exported to other rural communities, but also potentially scaled up to influence urban outcomes, there is a lot of opportunity.

The challenge is finding promising innovations. He said that less money is needed to make a difference in a rural community, adding "When I watch some of my federal partners, they think in terms of millions. I think in terms of thousands."

Turning to political considerations, Meit described the need to do a better job of communicating to rural residents the benefits provided by federal programs. "When the issues are framed properly, they support the activities that are being provided," he said. For example, with public–private partnerships, the private side of the partnership can resonate more strongly in rural communities, and he explained that "if our residents support us, they will communicate to policy makers."

Morris added that rural health and inequities between rural and urban areas have traditionally been bipartisan issues. Starting with the data opens the door to talking about the challenges that exist today, regardless of political party. Also, states, foundations, and other entities beyond the federal government have invested in rural health. "We can do a better job of connecting people to resources," he said.

Finally, both keynote speakers referred to the importance of transportation in shaping rural health care. "In every rural meeting we have held, the two issues that come out at the top in terms of infrastructure capacities are transportation and broadband," said Meit. Morris agreed about the importance of transportation, adding "Sometimes we make it harder than it needs to be." A Head Start van may not be able to transport anybody else because of liability issues. School buses can only transport students, and senior services transportation can only take seniors. "We can get more creative if we would just untie ourselves," he concluded.

3

Leveraging Resources to Advance Equity in Rural Areas

Points Made by the Speakers

- Many local and regional foundations are focused on accessing the resources that exist in a community, securing resources from outside the community, and using those combined resources to build on a community's strengths. (Lucky)
- The histories and cultures of particular places can be both obstacles and assets in working for change. (Browning)
- If people feel defeated by poverty, unemployment, and a lack of social support, their health is not necessarily their top priority. (Browning)
- Collaborations between foundations, businesses, and government can leverage the capacities of each partner. (Roybal)
- Rural communities can act as a microcosm in addressing problems that occur throughout the nation. (Roybal)

Foundations are part of a "third sector," beyond government and industry, that seeks to leverage resources to achieve the missions of its organizations. At the workshop, three leaders of local and regional foundations discussed the particular challenges of securing and applying resources to build on the community's strengths in rural areas.

THE BLACK BELT COMMUNITY FOUNDATION

The Black Belt Community Foundation serves 12 rural counties in Alabama's Black Belt, a name referring to the band of rich black soils stretching across Alabama that is well suited for growing cotton. The Black Belt is one of the most pluralistic areas in the state, said the foundation's executive director, Felecia Lucky. It is diverse in race, age, political ideology, and educational attainment. The Black Belt Community Foundation seeks to enhance this dynamic region by investing in programs and organizations that aim to bring communities together.[1]

Many African Americans within the Black Belt still reside in the areas where their slave ancestors once lived. The legacies of slavery have had and continue to have a detrimental effect on the lives of those living in former slave-holding areas, said Lucky.

The foundation originated when leaders and organizers in the region came together in 2002 and noticed that many philanthropic dollars were coming into the state of Alabama, but very few were reaching the 12 counties that needed them most. Instead, change was being funded by the people who lived in those communities, said Lucky. The foundation was established as a way of forging a collective stream of giving from the community and other sources so the people of the Black Belt can continually lift themselves up by "taking what we have to make what we need," she said. (This phrase gradually became a theme of the entire workshop.) It strives to create a flow of resources from the community, to the community, and by the community, coupling resources that currently exist in the community with resources from outside the community to create positive change. The foundation's vision statement says it this way:

> We believe that every member of our community has a vested interest in seeing our vision—a transformed Black Belt, where all of our residents contribute to healthy communities and reap the benefits of our shared gifts and a productive regional economy—realized.

The foundation's first task was to explain to the people it served what a community foundation is and does. Lucky listed the foundation's values:

- We place the community as our highest priority.
- We value the strengths of a multifaceted community where economic, racial, and social justice are universally practiced.
- We value relationships and connections that build trust.

---

[1] The foundation does not serve Montgomery County, in which the city of Montgomery lies, because it has a separate community foundation.

- We value integrity, inclusion, and transparency in both grant making and stewardship of resources.
- We value community leadership in acquiring and sharing knowledge.

"Those sound like buzzwords, but they are really words that we live by," said Lucky.

Its first grant-making cycle was in 2005, with a particular focus on nonprofit organizations that could help transform aspects of the community. The Black Belt Arts Initiative Grants Program, for example, provides funding to support nonprofits that promote the arts. The foundation's Community Associate Program (which is its signature grassroots leadership development program) has provided training opportunities for over 120 individuals throughout the region. The foundation provides capacity building workshops that cover governance, financial administration, volunteer management, and other tailored trainings to support grantees. Its community grants program provides support for a wide variety of projects, including volunteer fire departments and tutorial programs.

As a specific example, Lucky described Project United, which is a partnership between the foundation's community associates and the University of Alabama's School of Medicine and Rural Health to conduct research on health disparities in the region. The research is owned in partnership between the community and the university. The community must sign off on how and when the data are used, and community associates are coauthors on published papers. Community volunteers share the cultural awareness of those communities and their thoughts about what types of research should be done to address health disparities, said Lucky, while the researchers teach the community how to conduct research. "If you have a Ph.D. or a title in higher education, that is important," said Lucky. "There are others who have a Ph.D. in community. It may look different, but the value should be equal," she added.

Other people and organizations can help the foundation do its work in several ways, Lucky observed. They can identify networks of collaboration, resource sharing, and co-strategizing that already exist; creating something new is not always necessary. They can prioritize leaders and organizations that have the trust of their communities and the influence to get people to show up and speak out. They can also support southern community leaders and organizations that are able to articulate how identity, history, and politics combine to suppress the power and prosperity of their communities. The report *As the South Grows on Fertile Soil* by the National Center on Responsive Philanthropy in partnership with the Grant Makers for Southern Progress provides details on many of these opportunities.

Lucky concluded with the words of the poet Nikki Giovanni: "Take away our drums, and we will clap our hands. We prove the human spirit will prevail."

THE APPALACHIAN COMMUNITY FUND

The Appalachian Community Fund has a mission similar to that of the Black Belt Foundation, observed Ashley Browning, an educational planner in the Office of Continuing Medical Education of East Tennessee State University's Quillen College of Medicine and secretary of the board of directors for the fund. It works to build a sustainable base of resources to support community-led organizations seeking to overcome and address issues of race, economic status, gender, sexual identity, and disability in central Appalachia. Browning described the fund's vision:

- To work for the day when Appalachia's land, air, and water are safe from destruction and contamination
- Where the economy is stable, strong, and provides diverse employment opportunities for all people
- Where government and industry are accountable to human needs without exploitation of people and their health
- Where justice, equity, appreciation of diversity, and celebration of our common humanity replace racism, sexism, heterosexism, and other "isms"
- Where wealth and resources are shared equally
- Where all children grow up free from hatred and violence
- Where justice overcomes oppression in any form

Appalachia has a powerful history, said Browning, as does Alabama and many other parts of the United States. Entrenched and sometimes corrupt local governments and lagging public policy have not generated sustainable economic alternatives in the region. It has strong ties to the coal industry and timber industry, with a strong dichotomy between owners and workers. She added that racism poses a major obstacle to the ability of groups to organize within communities and with each other in a broader social change movement. Racism is communicated powerfully and often subtly in society, Browning observed, and it exists even in communities and institutions where people of color are not physically present or are a small percentage of the community.

People in poverty tend to engage in more negative health behaviors, Browning noted. Some health care providers may think that the people they see do not have an attitude of responsibility for their own health. But Browning pointed out that if people feel defeated by poverty, unemployment, and a lack of social support, their health is not necessarily their top priority. She explained:

> If nothing is getting better, if I am stressed and I can't provide for my family and I feel no sense of connection, I am going to be more likely to give up. . . . Patients aren't taking responsibility for themselves and aren't following the instructions of their doctors because they have higher-level issues to consider.

The Appalachian Community Fund seeks to find the people who have been either forgotten or lost in the system and empower them to create change and make their communities what they want them to be, Browning said. It strives to be effective, responsible, accountable, democratic, antiracist, and committed to developing leadership. It believes that organizations need to work cooperatively and respectfully with each other and be accountable for their actions. The organization provides grants to community-based organizations that are working to end racism, sexism, classism, homophobia, ageism, and ableism; promote nonviolent communities; and build organizations that are fair, inclusive, and democratic. It supports a wide range of tools to work for social change, including community organizing, coalition building, community education, training, cultural work, and advocacy. The fund addresses systemic issues of inequity and forms of oppression, especially racism, with the understanding that the methods used to unlearn racism can also be applied to other isms, such as sexism and ageism.

With the 30th anniversary of the fund occurring shortly after the workshop, it has been engaged in a deeper form of needs assessment than it usually does. It has been listening to communities about their problems. "Tell me what is going to work to fix it," said Browning, adding that "if we are on board as a group, the money is yours to go after it."

The following are examples of work that the fund has supported:

- Reaching 5,000 undocumented immigrants in Tennessee with information about using the Obama administration's administrative relief to avoid deportation
- Connecting chemical safety with racial justice at a summit of 62 residents, community activists, local government officials, academics, youth, and scientists
- Challenging and postponing a road project that would have destroyed Chattanooga's historic African American Lincoln Park neighborhood and its old Negro League ballfields
- Examining, with an interracial group of middle school students, the effects of urban renewal, gentrification, structural racism, and classism in their own backyards

The fund's grantees include Centro Hispano, a nonprofit organization and welcoming center for multicultural families in East Tennessee; Chattanooga Organized for Action, a nonprofit organization that works to initiate, support, and connect popular grassroots organizations for the purposes of advancing the local social justice movement; and the UUNIK Academy,[2] which is a rite-of-passage program dedicated to transforming African American youth into respectful and respectable African American adults. In addition, it has cooperated with the Nurse–Family Partnership program, the Office of Continuing Medical Education at East Tennessee State University, and child care centers in the region. The work with the university, for instance, led to a pediatrics education program that allows rural providers who do not have access to pediatric specialists to ask for assistance in treating their patients in rural areas.

"To have an empowered Appalachia, we have to first empower the individuals," Browning concluded. She added:

> Empowerment is what brought me to the Appalachian Community Fund in the first place. Being from Eastern Kentucky, my dad was a railroader and my entire family were coal miners. [When] I found other people who were like minded and had the same struggle that I did, it was night and day.

THE CON ALMA HEALTH FOUNDATION

The mission of the Con Alma Health Foundation is to be aware of and respond to the health rights and needs of the culturally and demographically diverse people and communities of New Mexico, to improve health status and access to health care, and to advocate for health policies that will address the health needs of all. The foundation seeks to engage multifield and multisector stakeholders, including the public sector, the business sector, and the private nonprofit sector, explained Dolores Roybal, the foundation's executive director. The foundation prioritizes building on existing assets and funding systems change.

The foundation is largely a grant-making organization, with a particular focus on culturally diverse rural and tribal communities. For example, Roybal mentioned a partnership with Grantmakers in Health to locally match funding from the Robert Wood Johnson Foundation for a state grant-writing assistance fund. One of the resulting proposals brought in $34 million to New Mexico to help plan the health insurance exchange.

A collaboration between Con Alma and the Kellogg Foundation resulted in a 2-year assessment of the effect of the Patient Protection and Affordable Care Act (ACA) in New Mexico from a health equity perspec-

[2] UUNIK is an acronym that encompasses five of the seven principles of Kwanzaa.

tive. The foundation has also partnered indirectly with The Colorado Trust to produce a report modeled on The Colorado Trust report *Health Equity and the Affordable Care Act* (DeLay and Walker, 2013).

The foundation worked with Hispanics in Philanthropy to create a funders' collaborative for Strong Latino Communities and the Latino Men and Boys Initiative, which resulted in awards of nearly $2 million to New Mexico nonprofit organizations. "Con Alma's contribution was probably no more than $25,000," said Roybal. "Again, it is through working together that we were able to leverage those resources."

A 3-year initiative called Healthy People, Healthy Places was supported by a group of national and New Mexico funders, with Con Alma contributing one-third of the funding. This funding expanded the foundation's work in health equity beyond ethnic and racial disparities to the built environment and food access policies, explained Roybal. It has made multiyear grants to the New Mexico Center on Law and Poverty Healthcare Access Project, which has been working to remove barriers to Medicaid or exchange coverage for low-income individuals, and to the New Mexico Community Health Worker Association to recruit, train, and mentor community health workers to assist with the certification efforts of the 2014 Community Health Worker Act in New Mexico, which allows *promotoras* to receive reimbursement through third-party payers for their work.

Smaller grants have gone to Prosperity Works, which leverages resources and invests in families by removing barriers and opening paths to opportunities through a child savings account, and Las Cumbres Community Services to increase participation in policies that address barriers to safe and affordable housing for pregnant women, children, and families.

As these grants demonstrate, said Roybal, the core values of the foundation are community self-determination, diversity, and preservation and enhancement of cultural and spiritual assets. The foundation's focus is health equity rather than health disparities, she added, with *health* broadly defined to include behavioral health, oral health, environmental health, spiritual health, and well-being. "Health is much more than health care. That is why we fund things like housing, transportation, economic development, et cetera," she said.

The foundation uses a shared leadership model. A community advisory committee, which provides community outreach and needs assessment, is involved in financial oversight, strategic planning, grant making, and evaluation. An annual meeting of the community advisory council and board of trustees provides an opportunity to discuss governance, legal, and fiduciary issues. "This is a truly integrated model," said Roybal, explaining that "we are community led and community serving."

Roybal discussed some of the differences between health disparities and health equity in the context of her foundation. Focusing on health equity shifts attention to the systemic issues that affect health outcomes. As the New Mexico Health Equity Working Group states on its website,[3]

> Health care is only a small part of what really affects our health. The choices we make, our behavior, has a large impact on our health. But, the places where we live, work, and play—our social conditions—affect the choices we make.

As Roybal said, "We believe that health equity is where everyone has the right to good health regardless of zip code or skin color."

One-third of New Mexico is rural, which is above the national average. It is a majority minority state, said Roybal, with a population that is about 50 percent Hispanic, 10 percent Native American, and 3 percent African American, along with other ethnic and racial groups, and it is becoming more diverse. It is the fifth largest state in the nation, and infrastructure is lacking in some areas. For the state as a whole, racial and ethnic minorities suffer higher rates of mortality and illness compared with other groups and receive a lower quality of health care, she explained. Furthermore, rural poverty rates are higher than in urban areas, which can increase disparities for minorities in rural areas.

Roybal grew up and still lives in a rural community that is predominantly Hispanic and Native American. "I did not know that I was 'poor' until I went to do my graduate studies at the University of Denver," she said. "We owned our own homes. We had land. We had a barter system. We would exchange a truckload of wood for potatoes or apples or chili. We were just fine. I think that sometimes these definitions . . . can have an impact on populations and on communities that is a bit misguided," she said.

New Mexico is grappling with many issues that are of concern elsewhere. Health care policy, Medicaid, and immigration are of particular interest to New Mexico and have been a focus of national discussions. The state's population is getting older on average, and rural communities have higher percentages of older people. Many grandparents are raising grandchildren, which has been an increasing trend across the country. "We are kind of a microcosm for the rest of the nation," said Roybal. She concluded with the following:

> That is an opportunity. . . . Rural communities are very resilient and resourceful and innovative. We shouldn't just be doom and gloom when we are talking about rural communities. We have strong values, in terms of being community based, family based, and intergenerational. . . . That

[3] See http://nmhewg.weebly.com/resources.html (accessed October 23, 2017).

is why we do all of our work from an assets-based perspective rather than a disparities perspective.

MULTISECTORAL COLLABORATION

A major focus of the discussion session was how to best collaborate with other sectors, including business and government. Roybal offered a story. When the ACA was first implemented, the Con Alma Health Foundation went to advocates to organize a multisector advisory committee, but advocates said that they did not want to work with government representatives, and when the foundation approached government representatives, they said that they did not want to work with advocates. In the end, "they all came because they didn't want to be left out. They all worked together. They came up with this outstanding plan that was a true blueprint," she explained. Even though they could not agree on a small part of the report, they agreed to disagree. Roybal said, "Alone, we get to move from point A to point B, but together and collectively we can move from point A to maybe point Z."

Browning said that the Appalachian Community Fund uses a system based on concentric giving circles. When individuals from a community identify a problem, a fund is established to which different organizations can contribute. These giving circles have greatly improved the sustainability of programs, she said. The fund is also able to provide more tailored grants:

> We are doing a technical assistance program for our 30th anniversary, where we are providing thirty $3,000 grants to applicants who need technical assistance. Three thousand dollars doesn't sound like a whole lot, but when you are talking about a social movement in Eastern Kentucky that can't afford a computer to mine data, that means all the difference in the world to them.

Lucky said that the Black Belt Community Foundation both approaches and is approached by other organizations. An early lesson occurred when a university approached the foundation and asked to partner. "Once we learned and saw our own value, we went to the Alabama State Council on the Arts and said, 'One of the things that we can help you do, because you are a statewide entity, is help provide you access into communities that you aren't readily serving.' Until we recognized our power, we didn't know to do that," she said.

The three panelists also, in response to a question, talked about their work with faith-based organizations. "In the Black Belt region, we have worked from day 1 very deeply with our faith-based community," said Lucky. For example, a recent project with young men and boys of color involved faith-based communities throughout the region. She explained:

> When you have churches on every corner [with] the ability to influence large numbers of people, we have considered it very valuable. We have had to use some different approaches sometimes to get the faith community involved, but it has been worthwhile and has yielded great results for us at the end of the day. They have become a part of our board. They have served on committees with us. They see themselves as a part of the infrastructure of the Black Belt Community Foundation.

Similarly, the Department of Health in her region has a partnership with faith-based communities in addressing substance abuse issues, said Browning, adding that "what better resource do we have to tell people that it is okay to be an addict and still attend church?" Churches can provide people with resources such as support groups that incorporate a faith-based component into their recovery. About one-third of the Appalachian Community Fund's grantees are faith-based institutions that are doing work in their communities. "The stronger we can make those relationships, the more allies we have to fight the issues that we are fighting," Browning observed.

Finally, Roybal said that her organization approaches the issues both structurally and philosophically. Structurally, it encourages fiscal sponsorships so funders can get grants to organizations that are not necessarily set up to receive grants. Philosophically, it values diversity of thinking. "We ensure that we have different opinions, including faith-based opinions, on our board, our community advisory committee, and our staff," she said.

4

Building Greater Prosperity in Rural Communities

Points Made by the Speakers

- Natural resources, human-made resources, levels of education, working-age populations, and economic diversity are all correlated with economic and employment growth in rural counties. (Lewandowski)
- Good school systems, strong leadership, access to leadership, and a high quality of life can attract people to rural areas, while a lack of adequate and affordable housing, a lack of available labor, and a lack of child care can keep them away. (Lewandowski)
- The availability of banking and financial services in economically distressed areas can enable people to access credit, build assets, and improve lives. (Bynum)
- Undocumented farmworkers need health care, legal aid, and other services as much as other people do. (Romo)
- In the Navajo Nation, elimination of a 5 percent sales tax on healthy foods and imposition of a 2 percent sales tax on unhealthy foods has encouraged healthy eating and supported community wellness projects. (Livingston)

Many factors contribute to the development of health disparities in rural areas, including economic, historical, and cultural forces. Four speakers at the workshop discussed several of these factors in detail, including community attributes that are associated with economic and employment growth, the availability of financial services, and incentives to purchase and consume healthier foods.

FACTORS AFFECTING RESILIENCY

Ever since the major recession of 2008 faded around 2010, the United States has been adding jobs, although the numbers have slowed in the past few years. Still, most states have more jobs now than they did before the start of the recession.

Alabama is one of six states that continues to have fewer jobs today than it did before the recession (see Figure 4-1), observed Brian Lewandowski, associate director for the Business Research Division at the Leeds School of Business at the University of Colorado Boulder. However, job growth has varied among counties in Alabama (see Figure 4-2). In 2016—a year in which the state added jobs overall—73 percent of rural counties

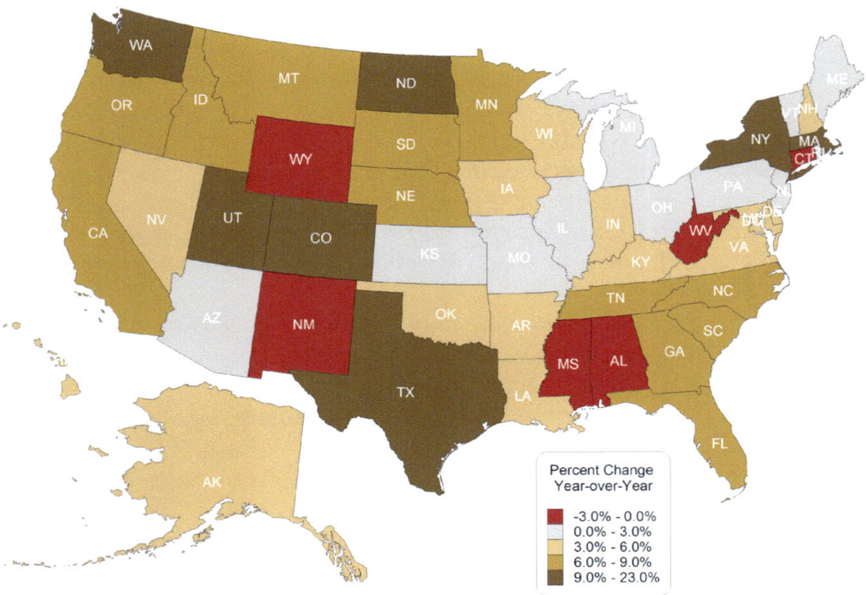

FIGURE 4-1 Six states in the United States had less employment in 2017 than a decade earlier.
SOURCES: As presented by Brian Lewandowski, June 13, 2017; adapted from BLS, 2017a.

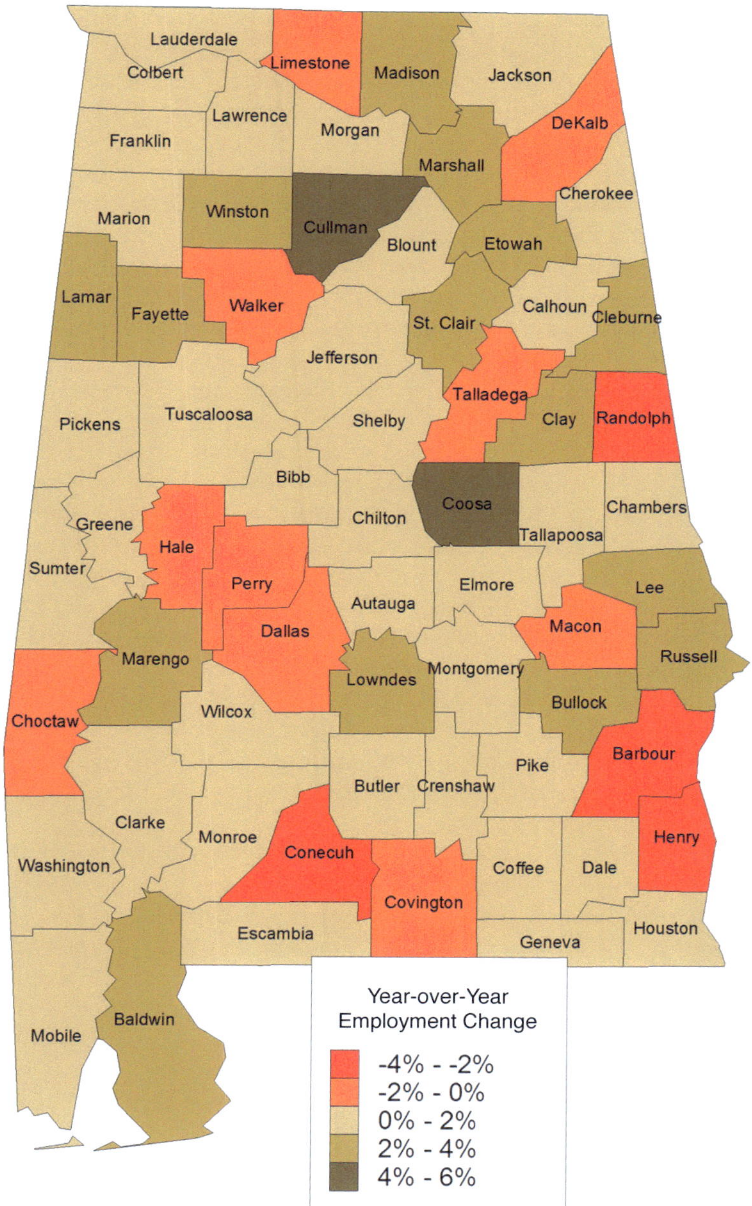

FIGURE 4-2 Fourteen counties in Alabama experienced declines in employment in 2016.
SOURCES: As presented by Brian Lewandowski, June 13, 2017; adapted from BLS, 2017b.

and 87 percent of urban counties added jobs. However, 14 Alabama counties lost jobs during that year.

As of 2017, rural Alabama as a whole has seen 51 consecutive months of growth in covered employment, which excludes sole proprietors, and employment is up by about 4 percent from the trough following the recession. However, employment is still 9 percent below its previous peak. The situation is somewhat better for wages paid to covered employees. Total wages paid in the state in rural areas are up 11 percent from the previous peak right before the recession, and average wages have been rising at a rate of 1.9 percent per year in recent years. However, annual average wages are still significantly lower in rural areas, at $37,400, compared to $46,500 in urban areas.

Lewandowski particularly focused on economic resiliency, which he defined as the economic performance of places after experiencing some form of disruption, from an economic downturn to a natural disaster. First, he and his colleagues sorted the approximately 1,900 rural counties in the United States from fastest population growth to slowest population growth on average over a 25-year period, breaking them into quartiles. Alabama has five counties in the top quartile for population growth over this period, and 40 percent of Alabama's rural counties are in the top half for growth. The other 60 percent of Alabama's counties are in the slowest half for population growth over this 25-year period.

Lewandowski and his colleagues then conducted the same analysis for employment growth. Only two of Alabama's rural counties are in the top quartile for employment growth, and only 25 percent are in the top half. The other 75 percent of rural Alabama counties are in the bottom half of national employment growth.

For the nation as a whole, rural America has underperformed in employment growth compared to both the nation and urban America. The same applies to Alabama, where employment in urban Alabama has recovered from the 2008 recession but rural Alabama has not. "Rural Alabama tends to get hit harder on the downturns," observed Lewandowski, adding that "rural Alabama also recovers less well on the upside compared to urban Alabama."

Although these statistics may seem discouraging, Lewandowski argued that "there are some things that can be done about it." A recent study in Colorado compared growth in population, employment, income, housing prices, and other metrics with a variety of economic metrics, including natural resources, education, and economic diversity. These comparisons provide valuable lessons that could be applied to Alabama, Lewandowski said.

First, natural resources tend to provide a competitive advantage for some places. A rich resource, such as fossil fuel development, solar energy, wind energy, or tourism amenities such as rivers and mountains, can be a source of growth. But many such resources are commodity based, and commodity prices are volatile. In an industry such as the coal industry, which peaked in 2008 and has been declining since, what was once a boon is now an economic detriment to growth because of this decline.

Human-made resources such as interstates, highways, community colleges, universities, correctional facilities, airports, and hospitals also provide a competitive advantage. For example, universities above a critical size provide employment and pathways to more education while also importing young people from outside the community, some of whom will stay and be part of the community. But those assets have mostly been built already, meaning that some counties have them and others do not.

The education level of residents is a powerful force for economic growth. In looking at Colorado's 47 rural counties, the percentage of the population with a high school diploma, a bachelor's degree, and a graduate degree was increasingly correlated with a county's employment growth. The percentage of residents with less than a high school diploma was negatively correlated with growth. "Education matters," said Lewandowski. Furthermore, this is a good lesson for other places because, as he explained,

> There are fewer barriers today for education than there ever have been. Not only are there so many campuses nationally, but through online learning we can continue our education without even having to leave our house. That is a positive story.

The percentage of the population between 30 and 64 years old is correlated with employment growth, implying that rural communities would be well served by trying to increase their working-age populations. Lewandowski has asked young people why they might return to the rural communities in which they grew up and found the following:

> It is appealing for some of them to come back. They reminisce about the area where they grew up. They want to replicate that for their families. How do you appeal to those people to come back to your community? How do you ensure that there is some sort of opportunity for people when they get there?

The percentage of a county's economy that consists of agriculture is also negatively correlated with employment growth. This could be because agriculture is continuing to substitute equipment for people, as it has been doing for many decades. It could also be that if much of the value added in a county comes from agriculture, the county's other activities are correspondingly weaker. Lewandowski encouraged counties to think about what kind of downstream product finishing they could do with agricultural products. If a product could be converted into "some sort of end user product before it leaves your community, that is a source of jobs and economic development within your community," he explained.

Finally, economies based on providing services have been growing faster than economies based on producing goods. Communities can work to build up their service economies, especially if they have access to broadband communications. For example, location-neutral businesses or virtual businesses can let employees and contractors live where they want, including rural communities. Similarly, while the tourism industry used to rely on the existence of hotels and other amenities in communities, the growth of VRBO and Airbnb has enabled communities to leverage the assets they have in ways they have not been able to before. "That provides another opportunity," he said.

Lewandowski and his colleagues also held focus groups in 20 communities around the state of Colorado to ask people what else mattered in economic development. They heard that health care matters, especially in rural aging communities where aging individuals want to make sure that health care is available to them. Families with young children also want to have local health care, and some rural communities in Colorado have been subsidizing hospitals to ensure that young parents do not leave.

Other factors that boost resiliency, according to the focus groups, are industry diversity, good school systems, strong leadership, access to transportation, and a high quality of life. Barriers include a lack of adequate and affordable housing, a lack of available labor, and a lack of child care. Of the positive factors, Lewandowski particularly mentioned local leadership:

> We heard many stories and anecdotes about critical individuals—they could be elected officials or they could be key business individuals or nonprofits—who have come together to help build something in their community. If it is putting away land for some sort of industrial complex for down the road for building, if it is building a trail along the river, if it is saving the railroad and turning it into a tourism amenity, there are countless stories where the communities that have been more successful in Colorado point to things that have been done in the past that are paying dividends today.

PROVIDING HOPE IN THE MID-SOUTH STATES

HOPE, which includes the Hope Enterprise Corporation, Hope Credit Union, and Hope Policy Institute, is a 23-year-old organization founded in the Mississippi Delta that initially focused on small businesses to create jobs that pay good wages and offer good benefits. "It didn't take long, though, to learn that the Delta needed a lot more than jobs," said William Bynum, chief executive officer of HOPE. Although jobs are "absolutely critical," rural communities need "the same things that communities anywhere need. They need health care. They need housing. They need grocery stores. They need access to basic financial services," he said.

Since its founding, the Hope Credit Union has evolved from a $1.5 million loan fund in 55 counties and parishes along the river to a provider of banking and financial services in three states. "We are a full-service bank, but we go where traditional banks don't," said Bynum. The Hope Credit Union uses every state and federal program it can and leverages policies that affect the communities it serves to build assets and improve lives in economically distressed areas in the mid-South.

A particular focus has been the need for financial services in communities where the poverty level has been greater than 20 percent for three decades in a row. Of the 384 counties that are classified as persistently poor by the federal government, one-quarter of them are in Arkansas, Louisiana, and Mississippi (see Figure 4-3). These counties rank poorly on almost every indicator of economic distress, including high-cost mortgage rankings, poor health, unemployment, and lack of banking services, noted Bynum. For example, all but one county in Louisiana and Mississippi that fall in the bottom quartile for health outcomes are persistent poverty counties. Counties marked by poor health outcomes also tend to have high minority populations. More than half of the 39 counties in Arkansas,

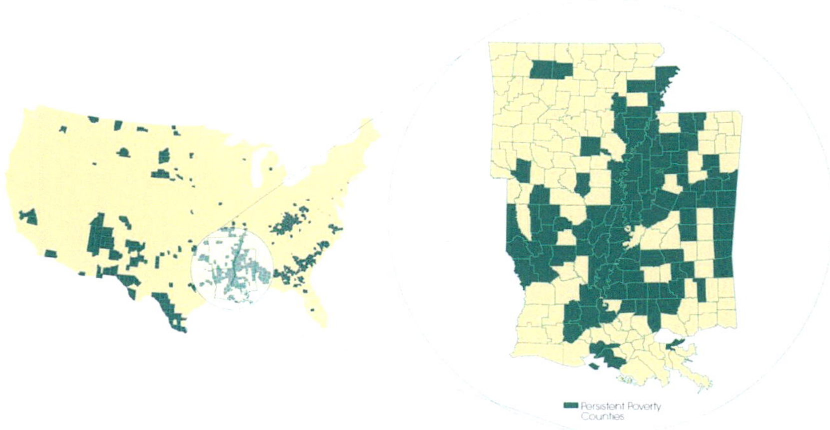

FIGURE 4-3 One-quarter of the nation's persistent poverty counties are located in the mid-South states.
SOURCES: As presented by Bill Bynum, June 13, 2017; Hope Policy Institute, 2016; adapted from Community Development Financial Institutions Fund, 2017.

Louisiana, and Mississippi that are primarily African American are also among the counties with the lowest health outcomes. Thirty-five of these counties are also persistently poor.

Housing affects health in major ways, noted Bynum. Homes that are not physically safe and that are either too hot or too cold put their occupants at higher risk of cardiovascular disease. Residents may not have access to grocery stores or places to exercise. Unaffordable housing can prevent families from meeting basic needs, such as nutrition and health care.

HOPE has worked hard to mitigate the burden of high-cost mortgages in the counties it serves. It is not a traditional bank, said Bynum. Its average mortgage is less than $100,000, and 76 percent of mortgages are to first-time home buyers, 74 percent are to people of color, 60 percent are to women, and 43 percent are made in low-income census tracts. Surveys of its buyers show that when they become homeowners, they are able to move out of low-income census tracts. "Homes are the primary asset that most Americans own. It opens up opportunities to send your kids to school, to start a small business, to climb the economic ladder. Housing is a core part of our work," he explained.

Bynum also talked about the ways in which health, education, and equity are intertwined. Greater educational attainment leads to better employment opportunities, which lead to better health. HOPE has worked with teachers and administrators in schools to provide them with access to basic financial services so they can better manage their own finances. It also received an $8 million grant from the U.S. Department of Education to finance charter school facilities. "I have mixed opinions on charters," said Bynum, "but it is a tool that is out there, [and] we want to make sure that communities that need education the most have access to whatever tools exist."

Mississippi has only eight counties where the unemployment rate falls below 10 percent for African Americans. In contrast, it has only eight counties where the unemployment rate for white residents is above 10 percent. In Kemper County, Mississippi, the African American unemployment rate is 20 percent, while the white unemployment rate is 1 percent.

Stress has a significant effect on health in these counties, Bynum reported. Laid off workers are 83 percent more likely to develop a stress-related condition, such as a stroke, heart attack, health disease, or arthritis. About two-thirds of the jobs HOPE has helped create through its small business loan fund offer health insurance to their workers, helping to reduce stress. "We don't intuitively connect health and jobs, but it is clear," he said.

Eliminating food deserts is another focus of HOPE's work. After Hurricane Katrina, New Orleans had the highest concentration of food deserts of any urban area in the country. HOPE worked with the city to create a healthy food financing program. A recent study indicated that the level of food access had returned to pre-Katrina levels and was more equitably distributed across the city than before the hurricane. The organization has now received resources from the Michael and Susan Dell Foundation to extend the experience in New Orleans across the rural communities in the three states.

Before they joined the Hope Credit Union, 40 percent of its members did not have a banking account. Yet, having a relationship with a financial institution is one of the most important financial relationships someone can have, said Bynum. It affects people's ability to build assets, accumulate wealth, and access credit.

Since the 2008 recession, the credit union has grown from seven branches to 30 branches, three-quarters of which are in persistent poverty census tracts. In one four-county cluster in the Mississippi Delta, another bank donated several branches to HOPE that it had acquired through mergers and acquisitions. In less than 3 years, the Hope Credit Union tripled the number of accounts that the previous banks had managed. Bynum described one new account:

> We opened an account for a woman who on her 100th birthday opened her first banking account, an African American woman in the Mississippi Delta. Think what it must be like to have to live almost a century before you feel welcomed enough. That is why I mentioned earlier about inviting people in. She finally felt welcome enough to be able to walk in and open her first account.

The credit union has also opened accounts for children. Data show that children are three times more likely to go to college and four times more likely to graduate if they have even a small account, said Bynum, adding "I can't wait to see what these kids' futures are going to be like now that they have these accounts."

Recently, HOPE worked with groups from other parts of the country to access unspent dollars in the Community Facilities Program at the U.S. Department of Agriculture. "We couldn't, by ourselves in Mississippi, make the case. But collectively, we were able to go to Congress, and they pulled a half a billion dollars out and made it available to organizations like HOPE," with the money targeted for community facilities, nonprofit organizations, education facilities, municipal facilities, and other resources, Bynum explained.

As many other speakers at the workshop observed, listening to the community is critical. "We are a community-owned financial institution. They hold us accountable. That 100-year-old woman is my boss. She owns the financial institution. She votes on the board. We listen to those folks," Bynum explained. Also, the more tightly anchored an organization is to the community, the more it will be able to meet the needs of local residents, Bynum said. HOPE has been working with local mayors, he said, "essentially playing the role of their economic and community development staff," helping them talk with local residents and make strategic plans.

"It is only through pooling our efforts that we are going to close the gap between poverty, health, education, housing—all the needs that exist in these economically distressed places," Bynum concluded.

RESILIENCY AND OPPORTUNITY: FARMWORKERS IN FLORIDA

Farmworkers Self-Help represents farmworkers in Dade City, Florida, and the rest of the state. Most of the farmworkers with whom the organization works are undocumented, but they need health care, legal aid, and other services as much as other people do. "They are a part of our big family in this country," said Margarita Romo, the organization's founder and executive director. "They do great work," she said.

Founded in 1979, Farmworkers Self-Help has, from the beginning, been based on self-reliance and resourcefulness. One of the first tasks the group faced was mastering English. For 7 years before the organization existed, Romo had served as a translator in farmworker camps. These camps tended to go unnoticed, as she explained:

> Most people didn't know that there were 15,000 farmworkers in Pasco County. Not even the governor knew that. When I began to call Tallahassee to find out what we could do, I remember one of his aides saying "Are there farmworkers in Pasco County?" I said, "Are there Cubans in Miami?" We still laugh about that when I see her.

The local college that Romo was attending gave the organization a room in which it could hold English classes. Soon other issues rose to the forefront. The group began working on immigration and amnesty issues, at which point Romo began representing the group in Washington, DC. The group "began to see how we could change the laws," she said, adding that "we started to find other people in Florida who wanted to do the same thing." The Immigration Reform and Control Act of 1986 "wasn't exactly what we wanted, but it was better than nothing," Romo said.

Farmworkers Self-Help trained and organized paralegals to process individuals and families under the provisions allowing legalization of immigrants who had entered the United States before 1982. The organization processed thousands of families and taught other organizations in Florida how to do the same.

It then turned to health care issues, working with other organizations around Dade City. "There are people alive today because of the organizing that we were able to do," said Romo. It began working with the health department and started its first *Promotores de Salud* program. "We learned about breast cancer. We learned about cervical cancer. We learned about diabetes because it was killing our people. We learned about hypertension. All of those things we began to teach our community women," Romo explained. The program provided information to farmworkers through clinics, hospitals, and partnerships with colleges and universities. "We have had to navigate our way through all of these things," she said.

The organization brought farmworkers to Tallahassee to speak with state legislators, which led to legislation providing legal immigrant children with health care without a waiting period. It also helped pass legislation granting immigrant children in-state tuition. Five young people who fall under Deferred Action for Childhood Arrivals (DACA) provisions have graduated from St. Leo University in Dade City, Romo observed.

Farmworkers Self-Help has done work to revitalize the Tommy Town neighborhood of Dade City, organizing bus service, a 4-H club, and a youth entrepreneurs club. Undocumented people are "part of your community," said Romo. "I am praying that we will have a way to have a new immigration reform so that we will be able to have more people free. They have already worked out there in the fields. They have given you all they have," she added.

"We all have something to share," Romo said. "Sometimes we have to shake each other to remind us of that, but we do have it. When we bring that out, it gives us hope that other people may not have," she concluded.

HEALTHY DINÉ NATION TAX INITIATIVES

The Diné Community Advocacy Alliance (DCAA) was formed in March 2012 in response to the high rates of obesity, diabetes, and the complications of these health problems among children, youth, families, adults, and elders living in Navajo communities. The alliance comprises grassroots-level community health advocates from various communities, with a mission of raising awareness, informing, educating, and mobilizing community members to combat obesity, diabetes, and other chronic health issues. In Navajo, the alliance promotes the idea of *shánah daniidlį́įgo as'ah neildeehdoo*—let's live a long life.

Healthy food is a Navajo tradition, said Denisa Livingston, a member of the Navajo Nation and a community health advocate for DCAA. But many Navajo people have been what she called "hijacked" by the unhealthy food industry. When the Navajo people were moved to a concentration camp at Bosque Redondo in New Mexico, they were given salt, sugar, flour, and canned meats to eat. "We are still trying to address that prison food," said Livingston. The Navajo Nation is the size of West Virginia but has only 11 grocery stores, so in many cases, people have to drive hundreds of miles each way to buy groceries. One out of three Navajo people are diabetic. "Every Navajo family is affected by this. This is the reason for our work," Livingston said.

The people she represents are eager for change, Livingston observed. They want to be seen as assets rather than liabilities. They have supported advocates like Livingston to make a difference in their lives. "Just as it takes a community to raise a child, it takes a community to raise a community advocate," she said.

DCAA has focused on policy and legislative changes. First, it has sought to eliminate a 5 percent Navajo Nation sales tax on healthy foods and to add a 2 percent sales tax on unhealthy foods. In 2014 these initiatives led to the elimination of the 5 percent sales tax on fresh fruits, fresh vegetables, nuts, nut butters, seeds, and water. Livingston explained, "The main area of this healthy foods tax law was to put an emphasis on our cultural foods . . . the foods that empower us, that make us strong, that strengthen us." Then, the Healthy Diné Nation Act of 2014 was enacted and took effect in 2015, which imposed a 2 percent tax (on top of the existing 5 percent tax in most areas of the Navajo Nation) on unhealthy foods high in salt, saturated fat, and sugar.

The greatest success of the legislation was raising awareness of unhealthy foods, said Livingston. Nothing in the Navajo language meant "junk food," so with support from the elders and Navajo language speakers, a new term was introduced: *ch'iyáán bizhool*, with *ch'iyáán* meaning "the scraps, the leftovers, the nonnutritious pieces," according to Livingston. The law imposed a tax on five categories of food:

1. Beverages: soda, energy drinks, flavored water, iced teas and coffees, fruit and veggie drinks, alcohol-free and alcoholic drinks, etc.
2. Sweets: candy, frozen desserts, pastries, cakes, puddings, etc.
3. Chips and crisps: baked, toasted, fried products
4. Fast food: ready to eat, quick, available, quickly served foods, canned meats
5. Flavor enhancers: salt, sugar, sweeteners

Each of these categories is defined in much more detail, and the places where food is sold are specified so compliance with the law can be ensured.

The 2 percent tax, through the first quarter of 2017, had raised $2.6 million, even with just partial compliance. This revenue has been going back to the communities through disbursement to all 110 Navajo chapters to fund community wellness projects, said Livingston. These community-based and community-owned projects address improvements to the physical and social environment of the community. Allowable projects include instruction, equipment, the built recreational environment, the social setting, education, community food and water initiatives, and health emergency preparedness. Specific projects within these areas might include developing biking and walking trails, traditional craft classes, healthy cooking classes, wellness workshops, horse workshops, and farming and gardening initiatives. Disallowable projects include meetings. The goal is to "allow community members to take control over their social environments and their physical environments to implement what is needed in their area," Livingston said.

In response to the argument that a 2 percent tax on some kinds of foods is a regressive tax, Livingston argues that the tax has progressive benefits. As Michael Pollan has pointed out, Livingston said:

> We can't afford the food that we are eating—the unhealthy processed food, the junk food, the cheap food, the oppressive food, the fast casual food, or in Navajo, *ch'iyáán bizhool*. We can't afford the heavy price that comes with it from the value menu. We can't afford cheap food because we are going to pay the consequences in dialysis centers, stomach stapling, health care costs, and unhealthy eating. It is something that we take to heart every day that we do our work.

The message has gotten through to the tribal leaders, said Livingston:

> They are eating more healthfully. They are buying more water. Our current Navajo Nation vice president, Jonathan Nez, runs marathons. It is changing the mindset, even in the leadership. Other tribes and groups around the world are considering similar policies regarding unhealthy foods, and the actions of the Navajo Nation can be an example for them.

An important lesson from the experience has been that community people can come together, increase awareness, and create legislation. "As community members, we are able to sit at these different tables with the executive branch and with these different departments. . . . [We] are changing the conversation," Livingston said. Problems and resistance to change will continue to arrive, and holding on to past gains and continuing to make progress will not be easy. But past successes have been "making a history for our future," Livingston acknowledged.

Livingston pointed toward several future objectives. One is to improve indigenous public health systems by using a model that focuses on community advocacy, tribal sovereignty, economic development, traditional food sovereignty, sustainable community wellness projects, community empowerment, and encouraging women to step into leadership roles. "For me, as a Navajo woman, my community and where I come from is a matrilineal, matriarchal society, where women are the ones leading. Yet, we don't see that reflected in our own government," she noted.

Another goal is to look harder for solutions to current problems through food. The problems are rooted in community members, and so are the solutions. CRAP (carbonated, refined, artificial, and processed foods) needs to be replaced with real FOOD: *F* for fresh fruits and vegetables, *O* for organic lean proteins, *O* for omega-3 fatty acids, and *D* for drinking more water. Healthy foods can help Native people reclaim their identity and change the narratives in their communities from being victims to being victors.

"Our currency was always produce. It was food. It was the exchange of these goods," Livingston said. "Our mindset of prosperity is also different. We are not only prosperous in having economic development but also spiritual health, cultural health, resiliency, and all of these different areas of well-being," she concluded.

INVESTING IN YOUTH

A major theme of the discussion session was the value of investing in young people to address inequity and oppression and to take advantage of the rapid changes going on in society. Working with youth is like "going to a different country," said Livingston. They are social media experts, whereas older people need to be shown how to work with technology. People in the Navajo Nation are very interdependent. If young people know they are part of a team working for a vision, everyone can move forward together to achieve a goal. Livingston particularly called attention to young mothers, who "know everything that is going on" through social media. They are "key people you want to reach out to. They have a lot of voice. They can spread the message and be a part of the purpose," she said.

Romo made many of the same points and noted that her organization is involved with camps where children can learn about social justice and with a theater group that has given a performance at the capitol in Tallahassee on immigration. Children "are our future," she said, adding "If we don't share with them and if we don't expose them to the wider world, they are not going to go there."

On a related note, the presenters talked about the potential of technology to alleviate some of the inequities in rural areas. Lewandowski pointed to the push by the Colorado legislature to ensure broadband access in rural areas. The last mile of connection "is the most expensive mile to complete, just as it was for roads and for electricity," he said, adding that "we are seeing subsidies and incentives for companies to finish that last mile. That is not only to connect households but, importantly, to connect schools." Broadband provides opportunities for businesses to locate anywhere, such as someone doing software programming out of their house or working for a company remotely. "We have even seen a trend where some companies are not recruiting people to a location but are finding people in a place and are building a remote office in that place," he said. A company in Boulder, for example, could find four people it wants to employ in Colorado Springs and quickly establish a remote office using technology.

Romo pointed out that the man who started the Youth Entrepreneur Students program for her organization is young and technologically proficient. "We have made room for a small office for him to have as much tech as he can bring together to teach our people and teach our kids, mostly. . . . This is part of the new regime coming up," she said.

Livingston observed that technology is a big issue in the Navajo Nation, explaining that "we normally don't have LTE or 3G. We have extended 1X. [Sometimes] you can't even send an email in a few seconds." At the same time, many Navajo also face more pressing issues, such as a lack of running water or electricity.

5

Equitable Access to Health and Health Care

Points Made by the Speakers

- Rural and racial inequities in Alabama contribute to substantially higher death rates among minority and rural populations. (Quinney)
- Anti-immigrant legislation and militarization along the U.S.–Mexico border systematically marginalize groups based on race and ethnicity, gender, and class. (Sabo)
- Community health workers can help create a common voice of action, engage community members in advocacy, change their own organizations to better meet the needs of populations, and engage at the civic level. (Sabo)
- Closures of hospitals in rural areas tend to affect populations that are older, poorer, sicker, and facing more barriers to receiving care, such as having transportation and insurance. (Thomas)
- Mobile clinics can provide primary care, including dental and mental health care, to children in rural communities. (Johnson)

Particular groups face unique challenges in gaining access to health care, which helps account for the health care disparities observed among these groups. Four such groups were examined in depth at the workshop:

minorities and people living in rural areas in Alabama, people living near the U.S.–Mexico border, people who receive health care from rural hospitals that are economically threatened, and children who live far from hospitals and clinics and lack ready transportation to those facilities. Speakers at the workshop proposed ways to overcome the barriers to care that members of these groups encounter, thereby reducing the disparities they experience.

INEQUITIES AND WAYS TO REDUCE THOSE INEQUITIES IN ALABAMA

"I challenge every audience that I speak with to get up and touch anything real that wasn't either produced in a rural area or produced using materials or resources that originated in a rural area," began Dale Quinney, executive director of the Alabama Rural Health Association. "We all need the rural areas, the heroes who live and work in rural areas, and the materials and resources that come from those areas, for our survival," he said.

Yet, these rural areas are facing difficult problems, Quinney continued. The age-adjusted mortality rate for the United States as a whole is 733.1 per 100,000 standardized population.[1] In Alabama, that rate is 924.5, the fourth highest among all the states. The age-adjusted mortality rate in Alabama's urban counties is 885.3, while in the rural counties it is 980.9, and in the Black Belt counties, it is 999.6.

Racial disparities also exist in mortality rates. For the United States as a whole, the age-adjusted mortality rates per 100,000 standardized population are 735.0 and 851.9 for the white and African American populations, respectively. In Alabama, those rates are 912.3 and 992.5. "Interestingly, the African American population nationally has a lower mortality rate than the white population here in Alabama," said Quinney, adding that "we have a very unhealthy population in this state."

One sign of an unhealthy population is a lack of population growth. Of the 67 counties in Alabama, 24, all of which are rural, had a smaller population in 2010 than they had had 100 years earlier in 1910. Five had only one-third of the population in 2010 than they had in 1910. Furthermore, population projections for Alabama predict that 41 of the state's 67 counties will decrease in population from 2010 to 2040. Quinney explained:

> What this means is that we are not having the economic opportunity and growth in our rural counties that we must have. Our children are going

[1] Adjusting for age removes the effect of age differences in populations.

> off for college or technical training or the military and are not able to come back home and have a career and be there around us when we get old and want them there and need them there. . . . This must be reversed.

In a previous position with the Center for Health Statistics in Alabama, Quinney helped develop the publication *Selected Health Status Indicators: Alabama's Caucasian and African-American Populations*, which compares the African American and white populations in Alabama and the United States on approximately 90 health-related indicators (Alabama Department of Public Health, 2013). The statistics reveal stark racial disparities, both within the United States and within Alabama. For example, with septicemia, Alabama's African American population has a rate of 26 deaths per 100,000 people compared to 17 for white Alabamians and 18 for African Americans nationally. For prostate cancer, the mortality rate among African American Alabamians was 59 per 100,000 people compared with 17 among white Alabamians and 37 among African American males nationally. For diabetes, the mortality rate among African American Alabamians is 40 compared with 17 for whites.

Quinney asked what steps Alabama could take to address health care issues in its rural communities. The first step he mentioned is expanding Medicaid. This would be an immediate step, as opposed to some actions that take longer to have effects.

Alabama should also expand the use of telehealth and telemedicine, Quinney continued. The state does not currently have parity legislation mandating that telemedicine be reimbursed by private insurance, as do Georgia, Mississippi, and Tennessee. "We need to be a leader in telemedicine rather than a follower," he said.

Rules and regulations should be changed to allow midlevel practitioners to do what they are trained to do, Quinney recommended. He recounted a call with the chief executive officer of a hospital in Mississippi that is near Mobile, Alabama, who said that the emergency room was staffed by four nurse practitioners from Alabama who drove to Mississippi to provide services that they are not allowed to provide in their home state. "We are losing out on quality care, especially in our rural areas," he said.

Alabama has a requirement that a hospital cannot be licensed unless it has 15 or more beds, which is a remnant of the days when long hospital stays were common. Alabama needs to change its requirements to allow small-bed-count hospitals in areas where they will not threaten the economics of other hospitals, said Quinney. The majority of hospitals in Alabama are already operating in the red, he said, so hospitals do not want others to be established that could further reduce their revenues, but small facilities could be authorized in places where they are needed.

Rural areas need help in economic development, Quinney pointed out, adding "I view geographical areas the same way as living entities. There needs to be a self-assessment of the area. Take a look at what you are good at, what you have, and then determine where you need to go in economic development." The Black Belt, for instance, still has its rich black soils, but much of its acreage is being converted from crops and pastureland to forests, which is a long-term crop that requires at least 15 years between harvests. "We need to look at the possibility of agricultural cooperatives to allow the small land owner in the Black Belt counties to get a piece of the pie," he said.

Churches, temples, synagogues, and mosques in Alabama have much to contribute in reducing disparities, Quinney said. "People trust the churches," he observed. "Members of the churches know the people in their community, even if they aren't members of that specific church, and will have them there for health educational events or screenings." Using a small grant from the Caring Foundation with Blue Cross and Blue Shield, the Alabama Rural Health Association is developing an online church registry where churches can register their interest in hosting health-related activities. In addition, electronic bulletin boards will allow churches to post notices for health-related needs while health care providers and trainers post notices for what they can provide.

Finally, the Alabama Rural Health Association is working with the Alabama Department of Public Health to establish county health coalitions that bring together hospitals, clinics, government agencies, physicians, nurses, mental health providers, public health officials, emergency medical services, the clergy, educators, and law enforcement officers to identify health care–related problems and possible solutions. Such coalitions can generate more funding from local, state, and national sources, said Quinney. "You are not just one entity. You are a voice of the entire community," he said.

A long-term solution to inequities is better education, Quinney concluded. People with less than a ninth-grade education in Alabama have a mortality rate two and one-quarter times higher than those with a high school education, and those with just a high school education have a death rate more than double those who have any college education. But better education cannot happen immediately, and many steps in addition to education need to be taken to reduce disparities in Alabama.

INEQUITIES AND WAYS TO REDUCE THOSE INEQUITIES ALONG THE U.S.–MEXICO BORDER

The U.S.–Mexico border region comprises 4 U.S. states, 5 Mexican states, 44 counties, and 14 pairs of sister cities that have much in common and work closely together. In Arizona, for example, the public health and academic sectors in the two countries have a long history of partnerships, and "despite what you hear on the news, we will continue to work together," said Samantha Sabo, associate professor of public health at the Center for Health Equity Research of Northern Arizona University. "We enjoy many binational projects at this point," she noted.

The U.S.–Mexico border is the busiest and most traveled border in the world, with more than a billion dollars' worth of goods crossing each day. In addition, Sabo pointed to six factors that together make the border unique:

- Ethnicity
- Growth
- Poverty
- Youth
- Shared infrastructure in health, education, commerce, and the environment
- Militarization

As an example, Sabo mentioned medical tourism, explaining that "when your tooth hurts, oftentimes it is cheaper to go down to the border and get your tooth fixed than it is to go to a dentist in this country." Another example is that Texas offers in-state tuition for Mexican nationals, creating substantial educational exchanges. Such exchanges can be expected to continue as the border population continues to grow, since at current growth rates, the combined population of the border counties in the United States and the *municipios* in Mexico will double in about 35 years. At that point, about 30 million people will live in the border region, representing about 5 percent of the combined population of both countries, she explained.

The population along the border is younger than the U.S. population overall. Latinos living in border counties are more likely to live in poverty than their state and national counterparts (31.8 percent versus 23.4 percent nationally). Children under age 18 who live in border counties (excluding San Diego County, California) are more likely to live in poverty (37 percent) than children nationally (20 percent). In 2012 and 2013, all four border states had lower rates of employment-based private insurance and the highest rates of uninsured residents, with Texas at 27 percent, New Mexico at 24 percent, California at 21 percent, and Arizona at 20 percent, as compared with the national average of 18 percent (United States–México Border Health Commission, 2014). In 2011, 29 percent of persons age 65 and under living in U.S. border counties (not including San Diego County, California) lacked health insurance coverage, as compared with 22.2 percent of their respective state counterparts and 17.3 percent nationally.

In the context of rural inequities in health, Sabo concentrated on the last item in her list of distinctive characteristics: militarization, which she described as pervasive encounters with immigration officials, including local police, and enforcement of immigration and border policy using military-style tactics and weapons. For example, during identity encounters, people are asked about their citizenship based on what they look like. Formal and informal checkpoints can pop up on the way home, to work, or to a store. People can be detained and abused.

Part of this climate is the result of anti-immigrant legislation that has been increasingly introduced and enacted in state legislatures. Such laws can discourage people from approaching social services, such as enrolling children in schools or visiting public health departments for immunizations. The result is cumulative exposure to institutional arrangements that systematically marginalize groups based on race and ethnicity, gender, and class. Such exposure can produce disproportionate vulnerability, stigmatization, discrimination, human rights violations, suspicion and distrust of state institutions, and deep disparities in morbidity and mortality among disenfranchised groups.

A survey of farmworkers who were predominantly permanent residents and U.S. citizens by naturalization or by birth revealed that approximately 90 percent of them saw border patrol agents on a daily basis (Sabo and Lee, 2015). These encounters occurred in neighborhoods, at worksites, at corner stores, and in supermarkets. Approximately 30 percent of the 299 respondents said that they had experienced some type of immigration-related mistreatment by a local law enforcement agent or an immigration official. Types of mistreatment included verbal or physical abuse, and racial or ethnic profiling. About 30 percent self-reported having poor mental health in the past 30 days, with smaller percentages reporting diagnosed depression or depressive symptoms. With any type of immigration-related mistreatment, whether experienced personally or witnessed, the risk of stress increased twofold.

Sabo mentioned stories of being detained face down on the ground at gunpoint, seeing the ladders on which workers were picking fruit being shaken by law enforcement personnel, and being placed in immigration vehicles without being asked for documentation. "These stories go on and on," she said, despite the fact that they are all permanent residents who have lived in this region for many years. She said,

> Their fear is deep—their fear of retaliation from the border patrol, their fear of losing their documented status. This is a real issue, because not only is there no place to go to complain about immigration-related mistreatment—the Department of Homeland Security is a very locked gate

> at this point—but even if there was, people are so fearful that something may happen to them or their families that they are choosing not to report the fear.

Building health equity in the border region requires listening and engaging in local response and resistance movements, Sabo said. An example is the Border Quilt project, which sought to express to the nation the need for revitalization and to memorialize the loss caused by militarization in the border region. Researchers, too, can use collaborative and mixed methods to listen, participate, and relay stories. The integration of statistical and thematic analysis can enlist Western and non-Western approaches to data collection, analysis, and inference to make sense of complex issues that no one method can grasp independently.

Sabo particularly emphasized the potential of working with community health workers, explaining that "they are lay leaders in their communities. They represent the socioeconomic, cultural, linguistic, and lived experience of the community members they serve. They have the pulse on most community knowledge." She has been working through a Centers for Disease Control and Prevention–funded prevention research center to be able to understand how community health workers, through leadership and advocacy training, can convert the participants in their programs to become citizens engaged in the political process (Sabo et al., 2013). Community health workers can help create a common voice of action, engage community members in advocacy, change their own organizations to better meet the needs of populations, and engage at the civic level, such as by bringing community members to school board meetings or zoning meetings. "Community health workers change the conditions within their communities," Sabo observed. They can "engage in various levels to take the voice of the people to the top."

Sabo closed by citing a phrase from a migrant shelter mural that she admired: "If we don't think differently, everything will remain the same."

THE CLOSURE OF RURAL HOSPITALS

The North Carolina Rural Health Research Program at the University of North Carolina's Cecil G. Sheps Center for Health Services Research tracks the closure of rural hospitals. It defines closure as the cessation of inpatient care, whether because the building is abandoned or it is converted to other purposes, including the provision of other health services. For example, said Sharita Thomas, a research associate at the center, a hospital might become an emergency or urgent care facility, an outpatient facility, or a rehabilitation or nursing facility.

Hospitals close for a number of reasons, Thomas continued. Contributing factors include the number of patients a hospital serves, management styles such as the willingness to take risks, how much charity care a hospital is providing, the types of patients a hospital is seeing, how profitable a hospital is, competition with other institutions, and the mix of sources paying for care. Whatever the specific reasons, such closures affect particularly vulnerable groups. Rural populations tend to be older, poorer, sicker, and facing more barriers to receiving care, such as having transportation and insurance. Race and ethnicity compound these disparities, Thomas observed. Furthermore, closures of hospitals are not regulated, so there is no way to know whether a need for hospital services remains in a community after a hospital is closed.

Since 2005, the research program at the Sheps Center has tracked 121 closures (see Figure 5-1). About 60 percent of these closures were abandoned closures, where no health services remained in the building where the closure occurred. In particular, Alabama has seen six hospitals close since 2005, of which four were abandoned closures. The hospitals that were abandoned served about 24 percent of the area's nonwhite residents, while the hospitals that were converted served about 18 percent of the area's nonwhite residents.

The majority of closed hospitals were in the South, which, along with the Midwest, has the most rural hospitals. These are also the states that were least likely to expand Medicaid under the Patient Protection and Affordable Care Act (ACA). Other studies of hospital health facilities have shown that closure of trauma centers, emergency departments, and public urban hospitals disproportionately burdens racial and ethnic minorities and Medicaid beneficiaries, Thomas reported.

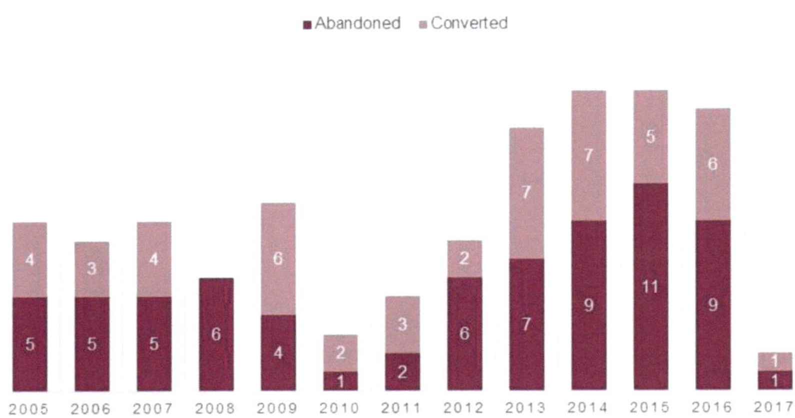

FIGURE 5-1 The number of rural hospital closures has grown in the 2010s.
SOURCES: As presented by Sharita Thomas, June 13, 2017; adapted from The Cecil G. Sheps Center for Health Services Research, 2017.

In looking at hospital closures since 2010, the North Carolina Rural Health Research Program has found that the rate of closures has increased from earlier periods. The closed hospitals tended to have lower levels of profitability, smaller market shares, and smaller populations to serve (Kaufman et al., 2016). Other factors may also have been involved, such as the percentages of racial and ethnic minorities in the population served, but they do not change the underlying conclusion, said Thomas. "We need alternative methods of health care delivery for these rural areas."

The research program also distinguished rural hospitals that were abandoned and those that were converted to provide some other type of health service. In addition, it considered the race and ethnicity of the populations affected, miles to the nearest hospital, and the community voice. A survey sent to city officials, members of the media, and health care professionals in the communities where rural hospitals had closed found that the community perceived the closure to have affected vulnerable groups the most, including the elderly, racial and ethnic minorities, people living in poverty, and the physically and developmentally disabled (Thomas et al., 2015). Survey results also revealed that transportation posed a major barrier to care after the closure of a hospital.

A more recent study compared 105 hospitals that closed to hospitals with similar profitability that remained open (Thomas et al., 2016). This study found that the markets of closed rural hospitals had smaller market shares, higher rates of unemployment, and higher percentages of African Americans and Hispanics. The implication is that rural hospital closures disproportionately affect African Americans and Hispanics, as has been demonstrated in other studies of health facilities. These results raise important questions about racial segregation and political power, health outcomes after hospital closures, and other methods of health care delivery, Thomas observed.

She also briefly described a case study of two rural hospital closures in the state of North Carolina. The Blowing Rock Hospital in the western part of the state opened in March 2005 and was converted to provide nursing care in October 2013. The Vidant Pungo Hospital in the eastern part of the state opened in February 2002 and was closed and abandoned in June 2014. Both had high levels of financial distress, including difficulties with financial performance, reimbursement, and hospital and market characteristics. However, Blowing Rock had both more people and a majority white population, while Vidant Pungo served a population with a higher percentage of minorities. The Vidant Pungo population also had higher needs, as measured by socioeconomic factors and health indicators. With the Blowing Rock Hospital, the community was involved early, grants were secured to transition the facility, and the closure process was transparent. With the Vidant Pungo Hospital, transparency was lacking, and the community did not know the hospital was going to close. "When it did, they felt like the rug was pulled from under them," reported Thomas. As one activist stated after the closure: "Vidant's leadership is immoral. You don't make $100 million and close a critical access hospital."

Thomas closed by touching on the accountability of researchers in doing these kinds of studies. "We are in a position of power with the research that we do," she said. "We have to talk about race. We have to talk about history. We can't default to someone else to do this." Health outcomes result from causative factors, which include geography and history. "We don't want to forget that," she concluded.

TAKING HEALTH CARE TO RURAL AREAS

As part of the work it has done for the past three decades, the Children's Health Fund operates more than 50 state-of-the art mobile medical clinics that provide comprehensive health care for some of the country's most medically underserved children. The clinics are "doctor's offices on wheels," said Dennis Johnson, executive vice president for government affairs at the Children's Health Fund and policy director for the Earth Institute's National Center for Disaster Preparedness at Columbia University. Most of the mobile clinics provide primary care, with some providing dental and mental health care. In turn, the Children's Health Fund has used its experience with the clinics to inform its work on public policy.

The fund supports rural programs in Arizona, Idaho, Mississippi, Tennessee, and West Virginia. Children's Health Fund programs in Florida and Nevada also provide health care in rural communities. These programs are informed by an adaptive learning process, said Johnson, with recognition and understanding of the full range and aggregate effect of factors that define the frame of health access in underserved communities. "We want to ensure that health status isn't undermined or interfered with and that opportunity isn't undermined for the kids who are poor and medically underserved," he added.

Johnson particularly focused on the need for transportation services, explaining that "mobility has always been a key consideration in developing programs to address access barriers. We were sending mobile units out to deliver health care." Other social determinants of health also had an influence on the program, including socioeconomic status, citizenship status, and cultural barriers, but "transportation was a big issue," he explained.

In surveys done by the fund, 39 percent of U.S. residents reported not having public transportation available in their community, and 11 percent of U.S. households were found to not own a working vehicle. While automobile ownership did not vary significantly by area of residence, the availability of public transportation did (see Figure 5-2). In

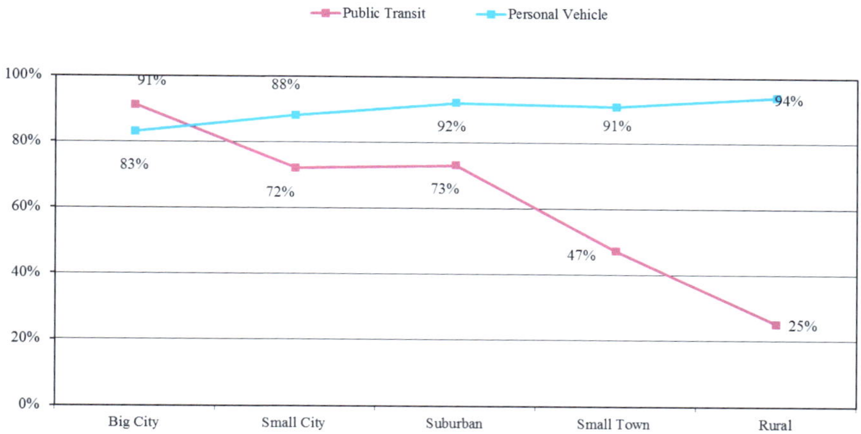

FIGURE 5-2 The availability of public transportation is significantly lower in small towns and rural areas than in cities and suburbs.
SOURCES: As presented by Dennis Johnson, June 13, 2017; Children's Health Fund, 2012.

rural areas, only 25 percent of people reported that they had access to public transportation.

Because of a lack of transportation, 4 percent of U.S. children, regardless of income, insurance status, or area of residence, missed a health care appointment in the year before the survey, including 9 percent of children in poor and low-income families. Of those who missed an appointment, 63 percent missed two or more visits during the year, and 31 percent of parents reported that they later sought emergency care for the condition associated with the health care appointment. Two to three million children in the United States were missing routine health care because of transportation difficulties.

This lack of transportation affects health in a number of ways, Johnson observed. It creates missed opportunities for immunizations and routine well-child care, increases the incidence of untreated chronic illnesses, increases the use of emergency rooms and ambulances for nonemergency care, and increases preventable hospitalizations. Medical transportation provider organizations must be committed to being part of the health care team to create a more seamless system and improve health access, Johnson said.

To quantify the severity of the issue, the Children's Health Fund developed the Health Transportation Shortage Index. It rates factors associated with barriers to primary care access, including area of residence, poverty (which serves as a proxy for not owning a vehicle), health professional shortages, safety net health care resources, and the public transportation infrastructure. It generates a score from 0 to 14, with scores of 8 or higher indicating where communities are at risk of inadequate health access because of transportation problems.

As an example of its rural programs, Johnson described the Idaho Children's Health Project in south central Idaho, which is affiliated with St. Luke's Hospital and the University of Utah Health Sciences Center. It serves a population of low-income, uninsured, and migrant seasonal farmworkers in south central Idaho, and the Children's Health Fund participates in the program through a dental health mobile clinic. Major challenges that the program faces are a lack of transportation, a lack of Medicaid providers, the geographic spread of community-based health facilities and the patient base, the growth in the permanent population of formerly migrant workers, and Idaho's rejection of Medicaid expansion under the ACA.

For the people it serves through the program and elsewhere, said Johnson, insurance coverage is not sufficient. Transportation deficiencies lead to suboptimal access to primary care and suboptimal management of chronic conditions. The result can be overuse of emergency care services, increased referrals to more costly specialists, increased health care costs, and poorer health outcomes. "The takeaway for us is that, in rural America, transportation access is the critical connective tissue supporting health access, opportunity, and ultimately equity," he noted.

Johnson closed with several recommended actions that apply both in Idaho and more broadly in rural communities. One is to monitor non-emergency medical transportation providers to ensure that they provide appropriate access. Educating and convening stakeholders could make them more aware of the ways in which transportation access affects health. Partnerships with hospitals, community health centers, and other human services providers could improve care, as could outreach to and engagement of state transportation officials in a meaningful cross-sector dialogue that fosters and enhances collaborative planning to better serve community needs. Involving local independent contractors, community colleges, and small businesses is good for communities and for people who need better access to health care. At the federal level, protecting Medicaid, budget support for the National Health Service Corps and Community Health Centers, and reimbursement for telehealth under Medicaid would all pay health dividends.

UPSTREAM STRATEGIES

The major topic of discussion during the question-and-answer session was how to prevent problems before they result in poor health outcomes. Sabo, for example, pointed out that social determinants of health are important factors in border communities. Community health workers are one way to address the longer-term root causes of health issues. But many members of those communities are dealing with basic survival strategies rather than focusing on long-term issues. "What will I do with my kids if I am picked up? Who is going to take over my mortgage payment? Who is going to take over my car payment?" she asked.

Johnson advocated working through some of the institutions that serve children and their families, including preschool, Head Start, and day care. He also noted that the Children's Health Fund screens for what they call "health barriers to learning," which are preventable illnesses that impede learning. Such illnesses as vision or hearing problems, behavioral health issues, and asthma can quickly be addressed. Johnson explained:

> If we focus on the front-end of children's lives and make sure they are optimally healthy and learning appropriately and not missing school, then we can take significant steps forward in terms of improving the likelihood that they will be healthy and well educated later in life.

This approach also empowers parents and recognizes the primacy of their role in their children's lives.

Johnson also called attention to the innovative telehealth programs that have been established for rural communities. The Center for Connected Health Policy has been tracking such programs at the state and federal level, he said.

Quinney advocated empowering other people in the trenches "to share ideas on how to improve things with those who are higher up." People who have direct experience with these issues have ideas that can be valuable. "There is plenty of intelligence out in the trenches. Call on it," he said.

Romo, from the previous panel, emphasized the power of educating people about health issues they may face, such as prostate cancer. Money is needed to do this kind of outreach, but funds for this purpose can be difficult to secure. "There are people in the community who make good teachers, who can take the information about breast cancer, cervical cancer, every kind of cancer, and teach it and share it so that we save lives," she noted.

The same approach is not appropriate for every community, Thomas observed, adding that:

> Senator Grassley has the REACH Act that is out there that is looking at different models of health delivery in rural areas, different ways to reimburse those facilities so that they can have the freedom to innovate and design a program that works specifically for their community, because it is not going to be the same for every rural community.

Innovations can also help manage the delivery of health care to the relatively small percentage of people who incur a large portion of health care costs while "maintaining our focus on the broader public health questions and commitment that we need to have to ensure that the public's health continues to improve," Thomas said.

6

Final Reflections

In the final session of the workshop, members of the Roundtable on Population Health Improvement and the Roundtable on the Promotion of Health Equity commented on the themes that emerged from the workshop, which are presented in Chapter 1, and on areas where further research, discussion, and action are needed. While not an exhaustive list, the insights and ideas shared by roundtable members capture both the progress that has been made and the many challenges that remain.

- Expertise of many different types is needed to understand the disadvantages facing rural communities, including the expertise of economists, geographers, and sociologists. All of them could be involved more extensively in analyzing the problems and potential solutions to rural inequities in health. (George Isham)
- Little information is available about the Asian/Pacific Islander population in rural America. Yet, groups such as the Hmong in California and the Marshallese in Arkansas are changing rural America and face many health challenges. The demographics and dynamics of many rural areas are changing, and Asian/Pacific Islander populations are just one aspect of those changes. (Winston Wong)
- The "three Es" at the heart of the work of the Roundtable on Population Health Improvement—equity, economics, and education—all need to be understood better in developing ways to overcome inequities. (George Isham)

- Rural areas are very different and require different approaches. "Coming here from California, I really have to remind myself—not only out of respect but out of humility—that we can't presume to have all of the answers for Alabama or New Mexico." In one rural community, a hospital that is struggling financially might be kept open even though people have the option of traveling another 20 minutes to a tertiary care center that offers a variety of services, such as a trauma center and a newborn intensive care unit. In another community, a hospital might close but then be used as a wellness center to improve health. (George Flores)
- Just as definitions of the term *rural* can be debated, the definition of *community* is not settled. Along the border, immigrants are not necessarily considered part of communities, and other marginalized groups can feel the same way. Strength and creativity originate in communities, which means that communities need to be considered holistically to maximize their capacities. (Octavio Martinez)
- Elections and voting are factors in inequities. "We didn't talk much about politics today, but they are the elephant in the room. Until we get better representation for communities of what they need in governance, many of the resources that need to flow to those communities will be absent." (Marthe Gold)
- People from areas of persistent poverty need to be elected to governmental positions so they can make a difference in their communities. "We have a lot of volunteers and a lot of people working in organizations in these persistent-poverty communities. . . . Maybe the next step is to do some training programs and get those community members to feel that they have an opportunity to be elected to government positions." Women's voices in particular have had a pivotal effect in communities and could be further emphasized. (Mary Pittman)
- If young people in rural communities can be engaged so they acquire the skills that contribute to the development of healthier and more prosperous communities, they will be more likely to stay in their communities and invest their talents in rural areas. "Civic engagement is a critical piece to cultivate at a very early age." Maintaining that, as well as education and skill building, will ensure that young people can help the community thrive in the future. (George Flores)
- The rural justice system can be a lever for change. Sheriffs, judges, and the juvenile justice system can have a large effect on health disparities, not only at a particular time in a person's life but for years into the future. Rural jails, for example, have a major influence on behavioral health. The rural justice system is becoming even more

critical given the opioid and mental health crises affecting rural areas. (Octavio Martinez)

- Despite the wisdom of taking "what we have to make what we need," money needs to come into communities to support education, or people will remain trapped in a low-education, low-wage economy. (Marthe Gold)
- Society is on the verge of profound changes, particularly as automation, robotics, and artificial intelligence change the nature of work and daily life. These changes could transform rural life, just as the industrial revolution did before. They will create "an opportunity to overcome some of the traditional challenges of rural sparsity [and] new problems." (George Isham)
- The most hopeful people at the workshop were those who were "closest to the ground and who had not left behind the people they loved." Mapping and acting on the hopeful and generative aspects of rural communities may be the best way to invest in the future rather than focusing on what is broken and how much worse some things are getting. (Gary Gunderson)
- A single person who gives voice to others can make a difference, even at the federal level. "I am leaving this conference on rural health equity with a good feeling about hope for the future." (Ned Calonge)

References

Alabama Department of Public Health. 2013. *Selected health status indicators: Alabama's Caucasian and African-American populations.* http://www.adph.org/minorityhealth/assets/MinorityHealthStatus2013.pdf (accessed December 13, 2017).

Bureau of Labor Statistics (BLS). 2017a. *Current employment statistics.* https://www.bls.gov/opub/ee/2017/sae/sae.htm (accessed December 13, 2017).

BLS. 2017b. *Quarterly census of employment and wages.* https://data.bls.gov/cew/apps/data_views/data_views.htm#tab=Tables (accessed December 13, 2017).

Children's Health Fund. 2012. *The health transportation shortage index.* https://issuu.com/childrenshealthfund/docs/chf_htsi-monograph__2_?mode=window (accessed December 13, 2017).

Community Development Financial Institutions Fund. 2017. *List of persistent poverty counties* [data file]. https://www.cdfifund.gov/Documents/PPC%20updated%20Oct.2017.xlsx (accessed December 13, 2017).

DeLay, S., and S. F. Walker. 2013. *Health equity and the Affordable Care Act.* Denver: The Colorado Trust.

Hope Policy Institute. 2016. *Persistent poverty counties in the mid South.* http://hopepolicy.org/maps/persistent-poverty-counties-in-the-mid-south (accessed December 13, 2017).

Ingram, D. D., and S. J. Franco. 2012. NCHS urban-rural classification scheme for counties. National Center for Health Statistics. *Vital and Health Statistics* 2(154).

Kaufman, B. G., S. R. Thomas, R. K. Randolph, J. R. Perry, K. W. Thompson, G. M. Holmes, and G. H. Pink. 2016. The rising rate of rural hospital closures. *Journal of Rural Health* 32(1):35–43.

Kretzmann, J. P., and J. L. McKnight. 1993. *Building communities from the inside out: A path toward finding and mobilizing community assets.* Chicago, IL: ACTA Publications.

Larson, E. H., D. G. Patterson, L. A. Garberson, and C. H. A. Andrilla. 2016. Supply and distribution of the behavioral health workforce in rural America. Data brief 160. Seattle, WA: WWAMI Rural Health Research Center, University of Washington.

National Advisory Committee on Rural Health and Human Services. 2017. *Social determinants of health.* Rockville, MD: U.S. Department of Health and Human Services.

Sabo, S., and A. E. Lee. 2015. The spillover of US immigration policy on citizens and permanent residents of Mexican descent: How internalizing "illegality" impacts public health in the borderlands. *Frontiers in Public Health* 3:155.

Sabo, S., M. Ingram, K. M. Reinschmidt, K. Schachter, L. Jacobs, J. Guernsey de Zapien, L. Robinson, and S. Carvajal. 2013. Predictors and a framework for fostering community advocacy as a community health worker core function to eliminate health disparities. *American Journal of Public Health* 103(7):e67–e73.

Singh, G. K., and M. Siahpush. 2014. Widening rural-urban disparities in life expectancy, U.S., 1969–2009. *American Journal of Preventive Medicine* 46(2):19–29.

The Cecil G. Sheps Center for Health Services Research. 2017. *Rural hospital closure tracking*. http://www.shepscenter.unc.edu/programs-projects/rural-health/rural-hospital-closures (accessed December 13, 2017).

Thomas, S. R., B. G. Kaufman, R. K. Randolph, K. Thompson, J. Perry, and G. H. Pink. 2015. A comparison of closed rural hospitals and perceived impact. Chapel Hill: North Carolina Rural Health Research Program. https://www.shepscenter.unc.edu/download/11685 (accessed December 13, 2017).

Thomas, S., G. M. Holmes, and G. H. Pink. 2016. To what extent do community characteristics explain differences in closure among financially distressed rural hospitals? *Journal of Health Care for the Poor and Underserved* 27:194–203.

United States–México Border Health Commission. 2014. *Access to health care in the U.S.-México border region: Challenges and opportunities.* El Paso, TX: United States–México Border Health Commission.

USDA (U.S. Department of Agriculture). 2017. Geography of poverty. https://www.ers.usda.gov/topics/rural-economy-population/rural-poverty-well-being/geography-of-poverty.aspx#datasource (accessed December 13, 2017).

Appendix A

Workshop Agenda

Achieving Rural Health Equity and Well-Being:
Challenges and Opportunities

Roundtable on Population Health Improvement

Roundtable on the Promotion of Health Equity

Montgomery Marriott Prattville Hotel and Conference Center
2500 Legends Circle
Prattville, AL 36066
June 13, 2017

Workshop Objectives

- Explore impacts of economic issues, immigration, and racial inequities in U.S. rural communities
- Learn about asset-based approaches to addressing these challenges

8:30–8:45 a.m. **Welcome and Opening Remarks**

Sanne Magnan, *adjunct assistant professor, University of Minnesota; co-chair, Roundtable on Population Health Improvement*

Antonia Villarruel, *professor and Margaret Bond Simon Dean of Nursing, University of Pennsylvania School of Nursing; chair, Roundtable on the Promotion of Health Equity*

8:45–9:45 a.m.	**Keynote Speaker Panel: National Overview of the Challenges and Opportunities in Rural Communities** *Moderator:* **Antonia Villarruel** *Keynote Speaker 1:* **Tom Morris**, *associate administrator for rural health policy, Health Resources and Services Administration, U.S. Department of Health and Human Services* *Keynote Speaker 2:* **Michael Meit**, *co-director, NORC Walsh Center for Rural Health Analysis; senior fellow, public health, NORC at The University of Chicago*
9:45–10:15 a.m.	Moderated Q&A with audience
10:15–10:30 a.m.	**BREAK**
10:30–11:30 a.m.	**Panel 1: Leveraging Resources to Advance Equity in Rural Areas** *Moderator:* **Ned Calonge**, *president and CEO, The Colorado Trust; member, Roundtable on the Promotion of Health Equity* *Speaker 1:* **Felecia Lucky**, *executive director, Black Belt Community Foundation, Selma, Alabama* *Speaker 2:* **Ashley M. Browning**, *member, board of directors, Appalachian Community Fund; educational planner, East Tennessee State University, James H. Quillen College of Medicine* *Speaker 3:* **Dolores Roybal**, *executive director, Con Alma Health Foundation, New Mexico*
11:30 a.m.–12:00 p.m.	Moderated Q&A with audience
12:00–1:15 p.m.	**LUNCH**

1:15–2:30 p.m.	**Panel 2: Building Greater Prosperity in Rural Communities** *Moderator:* **Bobby Milstein**, *director, ReThink Health; member, Roundtable on Population Health Improvement* *Speaker 1:* **Brian Lewandowski**, *associate director, business research division, Leeds School of Business, University of Colorado Boulder* *Speaker 2:* **Bill Bynum**, *CEO, HOPE Enterprise Corporation/Hope Credit Union, mid-South region* *Speaker 3:* **Margarita Romo**, *executive director, Farmworkers Self-Help, Florida* *Speaker 4:* **Denisa Livingston**, *community health advocate, Diné Community Advocacy Alliance, Navajo Nation*
2:30–3:00 p.m.	Moderated Q&A with audience
3:00–3:15 p.m.	**BREAK**
3:15–4:30 p.m.	**Panel 3: Equitable Access to Health and Health Care** *Moderator:* **Octavio Martinez**, *executive director, Hogg Foundation for Mental Health, associate vice president, Division of Diversity and Community Engagement, clinical professor, School of Social Work, The University of Texas at Austin; member, workshop planning committee; member, Roundtable on the Promotion of Health Equity* *Speaker 1:* **Dale E. Quinney**, *executive director, Alabama Rural Health Association* *Speaker 2:* **Samantha Sabo**, *associate professor, Center for Health Equity Research, Northern Arizona University*

	Speaker 3: **Sharita Thomas**, *research associate, North Carolina Rural Health Research Program, The Cecil G. Sheps Center for Health Services Research, University of North Carolina at Chapel Hill*
	Speaker 4: **Dennis Johnson**, *executive vice president of government affairs, Children's Health Fund; policy director, National Center for Disaster Preparedness, Earth Institute, Columbia University; member, workshop planning committee*
4:30–5:00 p.m.	Moderated Q&A with Audience
5:00 p.m.	**Closing Remarks and Final Reflections**
	George Isham, *senior advisor, HealthPartners; senior fellow, HealthPartners Institute for Education and Health; co-chair, Roundtable on Population Health Improvement*
5:30 p.m.	**ADJOURN**

Appendix B

Speaker Biographical Sketches

Ashley M. Browning, M.A., is an educational planner in the Office of Continuing Medical Education of East Tennessee State University's Quillen College of Medicine. She is a native of Belfry, Kentucky, and currently resides in Johnson City, Tennessee, after joining the university in November 2014. Ms. Browning has also held an adjunct faculty appointment in the Department of Sociology and Anthropology at East Tennessee State University since 2010. Since 2015, Ms. Browning has been a member of the Board of Directors for the Appalachian Community Fund and has been secretary for the board since February 2017. She also serves on the Patient Advisory Council for Mountain States Health Alliance, where she encourages positive hospital patient experience through effective provider-to-patient communication, and is a member of Kentuckians for the Commonwealth, the Alliance for Continuing Education in the Health Professions, and the Gay Alliance SafeZone program at East Tennessee State University. Ms. Browning's research interests include the role of social strain in Central Appalachia; the prevention, succession, and treatment of prescription drug abuse; and gaps between socioeconomic status and social goal attainment. Ms. Browning earned a B.S. in Correctional and Juvenile Justice Studies from Eastern Kentucky University in 2008 and an M.A. in Sociology from East Tennessee State University in 2011.

Bill Bynum is the Chief Executive Officer of HOPE (Hope Enterprise Corporation, Hope Credit Union, and Hope Policy Institute), a family of organizations that provides affordable financial services; leverages private, public, and philanthropic resources; and engages in policy analysis to fulfill its mission of strengthening communities, building assets, and improving lives in economically distressed parts of Arkansas, Louisiana, Mississippi, and Tennessee. Since 1994, HOPE has generated more than $2 billion in financing that has benefited more than 1 million people in one of the nation's most impoverished regions. Mr. Bynum began his career by helping to establish Self-Help, a pioneer in the development finance industry, and later built nationally recognized programs at the North Carolina Rural Economic Development Center. He is a member of the US Partnership for Mobility from Poverty, funded by the Bill & Melinda Gates Foundation, and serves on the boards of the Aspen Institute, Corporation for Enterprise Development, Fannie Mae Affordable Housing Advisory Council, NAACP Legal Defense Fund, National Committee for Responsive Philanthropy, and the William Winter Institute for Racial Reconciliation. Mr. Bynum previously chaired the Department of the Treasury's Community Development Advisory Board (as a presidential appointee), and the Consumer Financial Protection Bureau Consumer Advisory Board. A recipient of the University of North Carolina Distinguished Alumnus Award, his honors include the Aspen Global Leadership Network John P. McNulty Prize, Credit Union National Association Herb Wegner Award, Opportunity Finance Network Ned Gramlich Award, National Rural Assembly Rural Hero Award, National Federation of Community Development Credit Unions Annie Vamper Award, and Ernst & Young/Kauffman Foundation National Entrepreneur of the Year.

Ned Calonge, M.D., M.P.H., is the President and CEO of The Colorado Trust, a private grant-making foundation dedicated to achieving health equity for all Coloradans. Dr. Calonge is an Associate Professor of Family Medicine at the Colorado School of Medicine, University of Colorado Denver, and an Associate Professor of Epidemiology at the Colorado School of Public Health. Nationally, he chairs the Centers for Disease Control and Prevention's (CDC's) Evaluating Genomic Applications for Practice and Prevention Working Group and the Agency for Healthcare Research and Quality's Electronic Data Methods Forum Advisory Committee, and he is a member of CDC's Task Force on Community Preventive Services and CDC's Breast and Cervical Cancer Early Detection and Control Advisory Committee. Dr. Calonge serves on the National Academies of Sciences, Engineering, and Medicine's Board on Population Health and Public Health Practice and on the Roundtable on the Promotion of Health Equity. He is a past Chair of the U.S. Preventive Services Task Force and is a past member of the Secretary's Advisory Committee on Heritable Disorders in Newborns and Children. Prior to coming to The Trust, Dr. Calonge was the Chief Medical Officer of the Colorado Department of Public Health and Environment. Dr. Calonge received his B.A. in Chemistry from The Colorado College, his M.D. from the University of Colorado, and his M.P.H. from the University of Washington, where he also completed his preventive medicine residency. He completed his family medicine residency at the Oregon Health & Science University. He is a National Academy of Medicine member (elected in 2011).

George Isham, M.D., M.S., is a Senior Advisor to HealthPartners, responsible for working with the board of directors and the senior management team on health and quality of care improvement for patients, members, and the community. Dr. Isham is also a Senior Fellow, HealthPartners Research Foundation, and facilitates forward progress at the intersection of population health research and public policy. Dr. Isham is active nationally and currently co-chairs the National Quality Forum–convened Measurement Application Partnership, chairs the National Committee for Quality Assurance's (NCQA's) clinical program committee, and is a member of NCQA's committee on performance measurement. He is a former member of the Centers for Disease Control and Prevention's (CDC's) Community Preventive Services Task Force and the Agency for Healthcare Research and Quality's U.S. Preventive Services Task Force, and he currently serves on the advisory committee to the director of CDC. His practice experience as a general internist was with the U.S. Navy; at the Freeport Clinic in Freeport, Illinois; and as a clinical assistant professor of medicine at the University of Wisconsin Hospitals and Clinics in Madison, Wisconsin. In 2014 Dr. Isham was elected to the National Academy of Medicine. Dr. Isham is chair of the Health and Medicine Division's (HMD's) Roundtable on Health Literacy and has chaired three studies in addition to serving on a number of HMD studies related to health and quality of care. In 2003 Dr. Isham was appointed as a lifetime National Associate of the National Academy of Sciences in recognition of his contributions to the work of HMD.

Dennis G. Johnson, M.S., is the Executive Vice President for Government Affairs at the Children's Health Fund, a nonprofit organization that initiates and supports innovative pediatric programs designed to meet the complex health care needs of medically underserved, homeless, and economically disadvantaged children. Mr. Johnson is also the Policy Director, National Center for Disaster Preparedness at Columbia University's Earth Institute, where he acts as a liaison between the Center and policy makers and elected officials at the state and federal levels. Mr. Johnson directs the Fund's public policy, government affairs, and advocacy agendas and coordinates the Fund's relationship with a broad spectrum of public officials, public- and private-sector entities, advocacy groups, and health provider organizations. Prior to his current position, Mr. Johnson was the Vice President of External Affairs and Senior Director, Policy and Planning. Before that, he served as the interim director of the Fund's national network of mobile-based pediatric programs. Prior to his tenure at The Children's Health Fund, Mr. Johnson was a senior program officer at the Fund for New York City Public Education and a research analyst at the Public Policy Institute of the Business Council of New York State. Mr. Johnson received his bachelor's degree from the University of Pennsylvania and his master's degree in Political Management from the Graduate School of Political Management at Baruch College.

Brian Lewandowski, M.B.A., is a Research Associate Director at the University of Colorado (CU) Boulder and the Associate Director for the Business Research Division of CU's Leeds School of Business. He has been with the school since 2006, working on economic forecasts, econometric models, and market research and real estate studies. Mr. Lewandowski has a background in banking, international development, mining, and tourism, and worked for Fortune 500 companies, as well as with the U.S. Peace Corps. During his time at Leeds, Mr. Lewandowski has studied various subjects, including employment, industry composition, small business financing, exports, workforce, affordable housing, commercial real estate, film, government incentives, tourism, forecasting methodologies, nanotechnology, and others. He received his M.B.A. from the Leeds School of Business.

Denisa Livingston is a tribal member of the Navajo Nation. She is currently one of ten 2016–2017 Empowered-to-Serve National Ambassadors for the American Heart Association. She is committed to addressing the diabetes epidemic, the dominant culture of unhealthy foods, and the lack of healthy food access in the Navajo Nation. Ms. Livingston is a community health advocate for the Diné Community Advocacy Alliance (DCAA). DCAA has been globally recognized for the successful passage of several laws, the first of its kind in a food desert: Elimination of Tax on Healthy Foods, the Healthy Diné Nation Act of 2014 for Unhealthy Foods Tax, and a tax revenue allocation for Community Wellness Projects. From the University of Nevada, Las Vegas, Ms. Livingston received a bachelor's degree and a Master of Public Health degree. She is an alumna of Leadership San Juan and Leadership New Mexico Connect programs. She was a W.K. Kellogg Foundation nominee and a Slow Food International delegate of the International Indigenous Terra Madre event in Northeast India and Salone del Gusto Terra Madre in Italy. She is a member of the Slow Food Turtle Island Association, National Young Farmers Coalition, a national Sugar Action Group, and an advisory member of Reclaiming

Native Truth: A Project to Dispel America's Myths and Misconceptions. She was featured in *The Washington Post* live event—America Answers: Changing the Menu, *Gourmet News Magazine*, TV Tokyo, *Mother Jones*, Civil Eats, Al-Jazeera America, NPR, and others.

Felecia Lucky, M.B.A., is the Executive Director of the Black Belt Community Foundation in Selma, Alabama. The Black Belt Community Foundation was established to support community efforts that contribute to the strength, innovation, and success in Alabama's 12 poorest counties—the Black Belt. As Executive Director of the Foundation, Ms. Lucky values regular input from the communities and works diligently to strengthen the communities in environmental issues, health and human services, education, youth, arts and culture, and economic and community development in an effort to transform Alabama's Black Belt. Prior to serving as Executive Director of the Foundation, Ms. Lucky worked as an Internal Auditor in Minneapolis, Minnesota, and as an Accounting Supervisor in Memphis, Tennessee, for Cargill, Inc. Ms. Lucky then returned home to Alabama to serve as Executive Director of the Sumter County Industrial Development Authority. This position provided a tremendous opportunity for Ms. Lucky to effect positive change in her home county. With a sincere desire to improve the quality of life for Sumter County citizens, Ms. Lucky worked with Auburn University to spearhead Sumter County's first leadership development program (which graduated its first class in 1999). Ms. Lucky is very active in community development, serving on a variety of committees and boards, including Governor Bob Riley's newly appointed Black Belt Action Commission, the Southern Rural Development Initiative, Alabama Giving, and the Greene-Sumter Enterprise Community, Inc. Ms. Lucky earned a Bachelor of Science degree in Accounting from Tuskegee University. She also holds a Master of Business Administration degree from the University of Alabama.

Sanne Magnan, M.D., Ph.D., is the co-chair of the Roundtable on Population Health Improvement. Dr. Magnan served as the President and CEO of the Institute for Clinical Systems Improvement (ICSI) until January 4, 2016. Dr. Magnan was previously the president of ICSI when she was appointed by former Minnesota Governor Tim Pawlenty to serve as Commissioner of Health for the Minnesota Department of Health. She served in that position from 2007 to 2010 and had significant responsibility for implementation of Minnesota's 2008 health reform legislation, including the Statewide Health Improvement Program, standardized quality reporting, development of provider peer grouping, a certification process for health care homes, and baskets of care. She returned as ICSI's President and CEO in 2011. Dr. Magnan also currently serves as a staff physician at the Tuberculosis Clinic at St. Paul–Ramsey County Department of Public Health and as a clinical assistant professor of medicine at the University of Minnesota. Her previous experience includes serving as vice president and medical director of Consumer Health at Blue Cross and Blue Shield of Minnesota, where she was responsible for case management, disease management, and consumer engagement. Dr. Magnan holds an M.D. and a Ph.D. in medicinal chemistry from the University of Minnesota and is a board-certified internist. She earned her bachelor's degree in pharmacy from the University of North Carolina. She has served on the board of MN Community Measurement, and the board of NorthPoint Health & Wellness Center, a federally qualified health center and part of Hennepin Health. She was named one of the 100 Influential Health Care Leaders by *Minnesota Physician* magazine in 2004, 2008, and 2012. Since 2012, she has participated in the Process Redesign Advisory Group for the National Center for Inter-professional Practice and Education coordinated through the University of Minnesota. Recently, she became a Senior Fellow, HealthPartners Institute for Education and Research. She is participating in several Technical Expert Panels for the Centers for Medicare & Medicaid Services on population health measures (2015–2016), and is a member of the Population-based Payment Workgroup of the Healthcare Payment Learning and Action Network (2015–2016). She is also on the Interdisciplinary Application/Translation Committee of the Interdisciplinary Association for Population Health Sciences.

Octavio N. Martinez, Jr., M.D., M.P.H., M.B.A., is the fifth executive director and the first Hispanic to lead the Hogg Foundation for Mental Health since its creation in 1940. The foundation is part of the Division of Diversity and Community Engagement at The University of Texas at Austin. Dr. Martinez holds an appointment of Associate Vice-President within the division. He is also a clinical professor with an appointment in the university's School of Social Work and holds an adjunct professor appointment at The University of Texas Health Science Center at San Antonio School of Medicine's Department of Psychiatry. He currently serves on the National Academies of Sciences, Engineering, and Medicine's Health and Medicine Division's (HMD's) Standing Committee on Medical and Public Health Research during Large-Scale Emergency Events and on HMD's Roundtable on the Promotion of Health Equity. He has formerly served on the Institute of Medicine's Committee on the Governance and Financing of Graduate Medical Education (2014) and on the Committee on the Mental Health Workforce for Geriatric Populations (2012). From 2002 to 2006, he served as a Special Emphasis Panel Member for the National Institutes of Health, National Center on Minority Health and Health Disparities. Dr. Martinez also serves on the National Advisory

Committee on Rural Health and Human Services. He is the board chair of the National Hispanic Council on Aging, board chair for the Meadows Mental Health Policy Institute, and committee chair for the Texas Health and Human Services Commission—Behavioral Health Integration Advisory Committee. He is a Fellow of the American Psychiatric Association, a member of the American College of Psychiatrists, a member of the American College of Mental Health Administration, the National Hispanic Medical Association, the American Public Health Association, the Texas Society for Psychiatric Physicians, and The Philosophical Society of Texas. He has a master's degree in public health from Harvard University's School of Public Health, a doctor's degree in medicine from Baylor College of Medicine, and master's and bachelor's degrees in business administration with a concentration in finance from The University of Texas at Austin. He was Chief Resident during his psychiatric training at the University of Texas Health Science Center at San Antonio and is an alumnus of The Commonwealth Fund/Harvard University Fellowship in Minority Health Policy at Harvard Medical School.

Michael Meit, M.A., M.P.H., serves as co-director of the NORC Walsh Center for Rural Health Analysis and as a Senior Fellow in NORC's Public Health Research Department. Mr. Meit currently leads program evaluation and research studies focused on rural and tribal health programs, the national public health agency accreditation program, and health workforce diversity programs. He is conducting formative research for the Robert Wood Johnson Foundation to explore community assets to improve health and equity in rural communities, and recently completed a body of research exploring the impacts of health reform on state and local health departments. Mr. Meit has experience working at both the state and national levels, first with the Pennsylvania Department of Health and then with the National Association of County & City Health Officials. He served as founding director of the University of Pittsburgh Center for Rural Health Practice, and recently finished a term on the Board of Directors of the National Rural Health Association. He currently serves on the Board of Directors of the Maryland Rural Health Association and on the American Public Health Association's Committee for Health Equity.

Bobby Milstein, Ph.D., M.P.H., is the director of ReThink Health for the Fannie E. Rippel Foundation and a visiting Scientist at the Massachusetts Institute of Technology Sloan School of Management. With an educational background that combines cultural anthropology, behavioral science, and systems science, Dr. Milstein concentrates on challenges that involve large-scale institutional change and the need to align multiple lines of action. He led the development of the ReThink Health Dynamics model and a suite of regionally configured simulations that are used by leaders across the country to explore the likely health and economic consequences of policy scenarios. From 1991 to 2011, Dr. Milstein worked at the Centers for Disease Control and Prevention (CDC), where he founded the Syndemics Prevention Network, chaired the agency's Behavioral and Social Science Working Group, and was coordinator for a wide range of new initiatives. He was the principal architect of CDC's framework for program evaluation and published a monograph titled *Hygeia's Constellation: Navigating Health Futures in a Dynamic and Democratic World,* recommended by the CDC director as "required reading for all health professionals." Dr. Milstein has led several award-winning teams that bring greater structure, evidence, and creativity to the challenge of health system change. He is a co-founder (with Patty Mabry) of the National Institutes of Health (NIH) Institute on Systems Science and Health, and a co-developer of several other widely used health policy simulation models, including HealthBound and the Prevention Impacts Simulation Model. He has received CDC's Honor Award for Excellence in Innovation, the Applied Systems Thinking Prize from ASysT Institute, and Article of the Year awards from AcademyHealth and the Society for Public Health Education. Dr. Milstein holds a B.A. in cultural anthropology from the University of Michigan, an M.P.H. from Emory University, and a Ph.D. in interdisciplinary arts and sciences with a specialization in public health science from Union Institute & University.

Tom Morris, M.P.A., serves as the Associate Administrator for the Federal Office of Rural Health Policy in the Health Resources and Services Administration (HRSA) of the U.S. Department of Health and Human Services (HHS). In that role, Mr. Morris oversees the work of the Office of Rural Health Policy, which is charged with advising the Secretary on rural health issues. The Office, which has an annual budget of $147 million, administers a range of research and capacity-building grant programs that serve rural communities. Mr. Morris also serves as the HHS representative on the White House Rural Council. In 2012, Mr. Morris was the recipient of the HHS Distinguished Service Award, and in 2015 he was awarded a Presidential Rank Award for Meritorious Service. Over the course of his federal career, Mr. Morris has testified on rural health issues before the House and Senate. He has past work experience in the U.S. Senate and held various policy and program positions within HRSA and HHS. A 1996 Presidential Management Intern, Mr. Morris came to government after a career as a newspaper reporter and editor. He has an undergraduate degree in Journalism from the University of North Carolina at Chapel Hill and a Master's in Public Administration with a concentration in Community Health from East Carolina University. He also earned a Certificate in Public Leadership from the Brookings Institution in 2008.

Dale E. Quinney, M.P.H., is the Executive Director of the Alabama Rural Health Association. Mr. Quinney has a diverse history of working on projects as a health data specialist. He recently completed work in directing the development of a comprehensive statewide health assessment for the Alabama Department of Public Health. Prior to this role, he served as the Director of Statistical Analysis with the Alabama Center for Health Statistics from 1986 until 2000. Other past employment includes diverse data-related activity involving mental health, occupational employment, and unemployment going back to 1973. After entering employment with the Alabama Rural Health Association, Mr. Quinney visited every health-related facility, from hospitals to assisted living facilities, in 51 rural Alabama counties to learn more about local health care status and needs. Mr. Quinney was presented the Ira Myers Award by the Alabama Public Health Association in 1999. This is the most outstanding public health award in the state and is presented to those making a significant impact on public health in Alabama. He was again recognized by this association as a recipient of the D. G. Gill, M.D. Award in 2012. This award recognizes individuals for providing special technical assistance that positively impacts public health in Alabama. Mr. Quinney received his B.S. degree in business law from the University of Alabama in 1972 and a second B.S. degree in economics from that university in 1973. He received the Master of Public Health degree specializing in biometry from the University of Alabama in Birmingham in 1992.

Margarita Romo is the founder and Executive Director of Farmworkers Self-Help (FSH), a grassroots organization organized by farmworkers and former farmworkers in 1982 in Dade City, Pasco County, Florida. She organized AWING (Agricultural Women Involved in New Goals), and developed the Norma Godinez Arts and Education Center, as well as the Mi Otra Casa (My Other House) FSH community teen center. Through Ms. Romo's vision and efforts working alongside families of the communities that she and FSH serve, La Casa de Esperanza y Salud (House of Hope and Health), a free health clinic for farmworkers, has been in operation at FSH in Dade City since 1994. She is a recipient of the Robert Bannerman Award, the Clairol Award, and the Cramer-Fisher Award given by MAZON: A Jewish Response to Hunger. Ms. Romo is a past member of the Florida Education and Employment Council for Women and Girls, Pasco County Juvenile Justice Council, Pasco Arts Council, Girls Initiative of Pasco County, Pasco County Sheriff's Council, and Youth as Resources, Pasco County, and was appointed by the Governor of Florida and served for 8 years as a member of the Health and Human Services Board of Children and Family Services. Ms. Romo has worked with legislators throughout the years and during legislative sessions to effect passage of laws to improve the quality of lives of farmworkers and other poor. She has assisted in coordinating learning activities for visiting groups of teachers from poor areas of El Salvador, Peru, and Honduras. In 2013 she was selected by Florida Governor Rick Scott to be the first Mexican American woman inducted into the Florida Civil Rights Hall of Fame. In 2014, she was honored as a Public Health Hero by the Florida Department of Health. In April 2015 Ms. Romo was awarded the 2015 Sapphire Award in the Individual Category from the Blue Foundation of Blue Cross Blue Shield of Florida. Also in April 2015, Ms. Romo received the Honorary Doctorate of Humane Letters at St. Leo University in San Antonio, Florida. In November 2015 Ms. Romo received the Lightning Community Hero Award from the Tampa Bay Lightning Foundation. She continues to travel to the state capitol in Tallahassee and to Congress and other venues across Florida and the country and works tirelessly against poverty and prejudice.

Dolores E. Roybal, Ph.D., M.S.W., is the executive director of Con Alma Health Foundation, the largest foundation in New Mexico dedicated solely to health. Con Alma's mission is to be aware of and address the health rights and needs of the culturally and demographically diverse peoples and communities of New Mexico with a focus on rural, tribal, and communities of color. A health equity foundation, Con Alma was recently awarded the Public Health Advocate Award for "an organization that has made a positive health-related change in their community" from the New Mexico Public Health Association. A native New Mexican, Dr. Roybal has more than 35 years of experience in nonprofit and philanthropy work. She currently serves as a board member of the Border Philanthropy Partnership, a binational organization, and as a former board member and chair of the New Mexico Association of Grantmakers, Grantmakers In Health, and Hispanics in Philanthropy. Prior positions include program director at the Santa Fe Community Foundation, founding executive director of NGO NM, a statewide nonprofit association, and executive director of Women's Health Services. She also directed Graduate and External Programs at the College of Santa Fe, and served as the graduate Social Work coordinator at New Mexico Highlands University. She has taught both graduate and undergraduate courses for many years. She has a master's in social work and a Ph.D. in organizational behavior and development with a focus on nonprofit management, philanthropy, and the nonprofit sector.

Samantha J. Sabo, Dr.P.H., M.P.H., is an Associate Professor of Public Health with the Northern Arizona University, Center for Health Equity Research, and affiliate faculty with the Zuckerman College of Public Health, University of Arizona. Her work examines the role and impact of community health worker (CHW) interventions and advocacy on chronic disease and maternal and child health disparities in diverse communities, including Latino, immigrant, migrant, and agricultural worker populations of the U.S.–Mexico border and northern Mexico. She has recently begun to partner with indigenous citizens, including traditional healers of the U.S. Southwest, to advance health equity. She prioritizes innovation in research, advocacy, and policy through community-based and participatory action research methods such as CHWs as researchers, mixed use of qualitative and quantitative methods, critical race and decolonizing research methodologies that include collaborative analysis, use of oral history, digital storytelling, and Photo Voice. Prior to joining the faculty, Dr. Sabo served as a Fellow to the U.S.–México Border Health Commission and later the Director for Transborder Initiatives (2007–2014), where she cultivated academic and institutional partnerships to facilitate applied public health research and public health workforce development in the U.S.–Mexico border region, including Mexico. In 2013, she co-founded a statewide coalition of more than 150 agencies to advance the CHW workforce and facilitate stakeholder engagement to shape research, training, and policy agendas and has scaled this work to co-found a large-scale effort to engage Arizona's 22 Tribal CHW programs in workforce development and policy efforts. She has been recognized for her commitment to community engagement, advocacy for social justice, and excellence in migration research. She currently serves as the Multiple Principal Investigator of a National Institutes of Health/National Heart, Lung, and Blood Institute R01 implementation science initiative to improve chronic disease outcomes among Mexican nationals living at the U.S.–Mexico border.

Sharita Thomas, M.P.P., received her Master's of Public Policy, with a focus in Health Policy, from the Sanford School of Public Policy at Duke University. She is a research associate with the North Carolina Rural Health Research Program. Her professional health policy experience is rooted in past work as a legislative or research assistant with the House Ways and Means Subcommittee on Health, the North Carolina Department of Health and Human Services, and the North Carolina General Assembly. Her focus with the NC Rural Health Research Program is managing rural health projects, especially work with hospital closures. Her other rural health project interests include social determinants, maternal–child health, qualitative research, and health inequities.

Antonia M. Villarruel, Ph.D., R.N., FAAN, is the Margaret Bond Simon Dean of Nursing at the University of Pennsylvania School of Nursing and Director of the School's World Health Organization Collaborating Center for Nursing and Midwifery Leadership. As a bilingual and bicultural nurse researcher, Dr. Villarruel has extensive research and practice experience with diverse Latino and Mexican populations and communities, and health promotion and health disparities research and practice. She incorporates a community-based participatory approach to her research. Specifically, her research focuses on the development and testing of interventions to reduce sexual risk behaviors among Mexican and Latino youth. She has been the principal investigator and co-principal investigator of more than eight randomized clinical trials concerned with reducing sexual and other risk behaviors. As part of this program of research, she developed an efficacious program to reduce sexual risk behavior among Latino youth titled *Cuídate!* The program is disseminated nationally by the Centers for Disease Control and Prevention (CDC) as part of their Diffusion of Evidence-Based Interventions program and the Office of Adolescent Health. In addition to her research, Dr. Villarruel has assumed leadership in many national and local organizations. She is the past President and founding member of the National Coalition of Ethnic Minority Nursing Associations and past President of the National Association of Hispanic Nurses. She has served as a member of the Health Resources and Services Administration (HRSA)/CDC HIV/STD Advisory Council, the HRSA National Advisory Council for Nursing Education and Practice, Health and Medicine Division Board on Population Health and Public Health Practice, and also as a charter member of the Secretary of the Department of Health and Human Services' Advisory Council on Minority Health and Health Disparities. She is a member of the Strategic Advisory Council of the AARP/Robert Wood Johnson Foundation Center for Health Policy Future of Nursing Campaign for Action and co-chairs the Diversity Steering Committee. She is also the chair of the Health and Medicine Division Roundtable on the Promotion of Health Equity. She has received numerous honors and awards, including membership in the National Academy of Medicine and selection as a Fellow in the American Academy of Nursing.